Problems in
Respiratory Medicine

Problems in Practice Series

PROBLEMS IN ARTHRITIS AND RHEUMATISM – *D. N. Golding*
PROBLEMS IN CARDIOLOGY – *C. F. P. Wharton*
PROBLEMS IN GASTROENTEROLOGY – *M. Lancaster-Smith* and *K. Williams*
PROBLEMS IN GERIATRIC MEDICINE – *A. Martin*
PROBLEMS IN GYNAECOLOGY – *E. P. W. Tatford*
PROBLEMS IN OPHTHALMOLOGY – *M. G. Glasspool*
PROBLEMS IN OTOLARYNGOLOGY – *P. Ratnesar*
PROBLEMS IN PAEDIATRICS – *J. Hood*
PROBLEMS IN PERIPHERAL VASCULAR DISEASE – *K. Williams*
PROBLEMS IN RESPIRATORY MEDICINE – *P. Forgacs*
PROBLEMS IN SOCIAL CARE – *J. Mogridge*
SERIES INDEX VOLUME

Problems in Practice Series

Series Editors : J.Fry K.Williams M.Lancaster-Smith

Problems
in
Respiratory
Medicine

Paul Forgacs
MD, FRCP

Honorary Consultant in Respiratory Medicine
Brook General Hospital, London

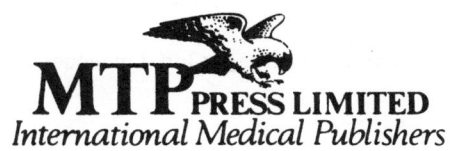

MTP PRESS LIMITED
International Medical Publishers

Published by
MTP Press Limited
Falcon House
Lancaster, England

Copyright © 1981 P. Forgacs
Softcover reprint of the hardcover 1st edition 1981

First published 1981

ISBN-13: 978-94-011-7220-2   e-ISBN-13: 978-94-011-7218-9
DOI: 10.1007/978-94-011-7218-9

Typeset by Swiftpages Ltd, Liverpool

Contents

Preface   7

Series Foreword   *J. P. Horder OBE*   9

1   Symptoms, clinical signs and breathing tests   11
Cough – Sputum – Haemoptysis – Dyspnoea – Pain – Percussion – Auscultation – Clubbing of the fingers – Cyanosis – Pursed-lip breathing

2   Pneumonia   35
Defences of the lung – Factors predisposing to infection – Classification – Clinical features – Investigations – Complications – Recurrent pneumonia – Differential diagnosis – Treatment

3   Chronic bronchitis   53
Prevalence – Pathology – Clinical features – Investigations – Differential diagnosis – Complications – Treatment

4   Asthma   69
Pathogenesis – Classification – Clinical features – Investigations – Differential diagnosis – Prognosis – Treatment

5   Tuberculosis   87
Mortality – Natural history – Presentation – Diagnostic tests – Investigation of contacts – Prevention – Treatment

6   Cancer of the lung   105
Mortality – Aetiology – Classification – Presentation –
Clinicalsigns – Progress – Investigations – Differential
diagnosis – Prevention – Treatment

7   Pleural effusions   119
Aetiology – Investigations – Differential diagnosis –
Tumours of the pleura – Complications – Treatment

8   Recurrent respiratory illness in children   131
Viral infections – Cystic fibrosis – Immune deficiencies
– Bronchiectasis

9   Fibrosing alveolitis   135
Diagnosis – Treatment

10   Spontaneous pneumothorax   139
Pathogenesis – Symptoms and signs – Treatment

11   Pulmonary sarcoidosis   143
Natural history – Treatment

Further reading   147

Index   149

Preface

The topics chosen for discussion represent the most common problems referred by family doctors to chest clinics. It was taken for granted that the reader will be familiar with the symptoms, signs, and natural history of respiratory diseases, so that the stress is on differential diagnosis and treatment.

Tuberculosis once occupied nearly all the time of chest physicians. At present weeks go by without a single case presenting itself. There has been no comparable improvement in cancer of the lung, which remains one of the most intractable problems. Asthma was seldom referred to out-patient clinics when the disease was regarded as more unpleasant than dangerous. The hazards of severe attacks and the advantages of liaison with a hospital department are now widely recognized. A similar change of attitude to the management of chronic bronchitis brought many new patients to the chest clinics in place of the vanishing tuberculous population.

Some uncommon pulmonary diseases are included: allergic alveolitis, because of the importance of early diagnosis, and sarcoidosis in order to discourage unnecessary treatment.

The book is intended to be a practical guide and is not a critical review. This might serve as an excuse for its didactic style and the exclusion of controversial subjects. Some statements are repeated at more than one place in order to help readers who wish to consult individual chapters bearing on some current problem. Source references are omitted and are replaced by a short list of books recommended for further reading.

Series Foreword

This series of books is designed to help general practitioners. So are other books. What is unusual in this instance is their collective authorship; they are written by specialists working at district general hospitals. The writers derive their own experience from a range of cases less highly selected than those on which textbooks are traditionally based. They are also in a good position to pick out topics which they see creating difficulties for the practitioners of their district, whose personal capacities are familiar to them; and to concentrate on contexts where mistakes are most likely to occur. They are all well-accustomed to working in consultation.

All the authors write from hospital experience and from the viewpoint of their specialty. There are, therefore, matters important to family practice which should be sought not within this series, but elsewhere. Within the series much practical and useful advice is to be found with which the general practitioner can compare his existing performance and build in new ideas and improved techniques.

These books are attractively produced and I recommend them.

J. P. Horder OBE
President, The Royal College
of General Practitioners

1 Symptoms, clinical signs and breathing tests

SYMPTOMS

Cough – Sputum – Haemoptysis – Dyspnoea – Pain

Cough

The clinical significance of cough as a presenting symptom of chronic lung disease is obscured by the vast number of smokers with mild tracheobronchitis and the high prevalence of common viral respiratory infections. Cough is often regarded as a trivial complaint and is not reported or investigated until it has persisted for some weeks.

In acute respiratory infections the cough usually clears up within 2–3 weeks. If it persists longer than a month it merits a chest X-ray, but is not necessarily a symptom of serious disease.

Irritable bronchus Following viral infections, particularly influenza, the bronchi may remain abnormally sensitive to inhaled irritants. Smoke, dust or cold air continue to trigger fits of coughing for several weeks after the acute illness. The cough may also continue for weeks after pertussis and in allergic bronchitis. Tumour Even so it is unwise to attribute a persistent unproductive cough to bronchial hypersensitivity until the possibility of an intrabronchial tumour has been excluded.

Acoustic features Cough is a forced expiration, interrupted by repeated closure of the glottis. In a dry cough only the expiratory breath sounds are heard between the sequence of explosive glottic

11

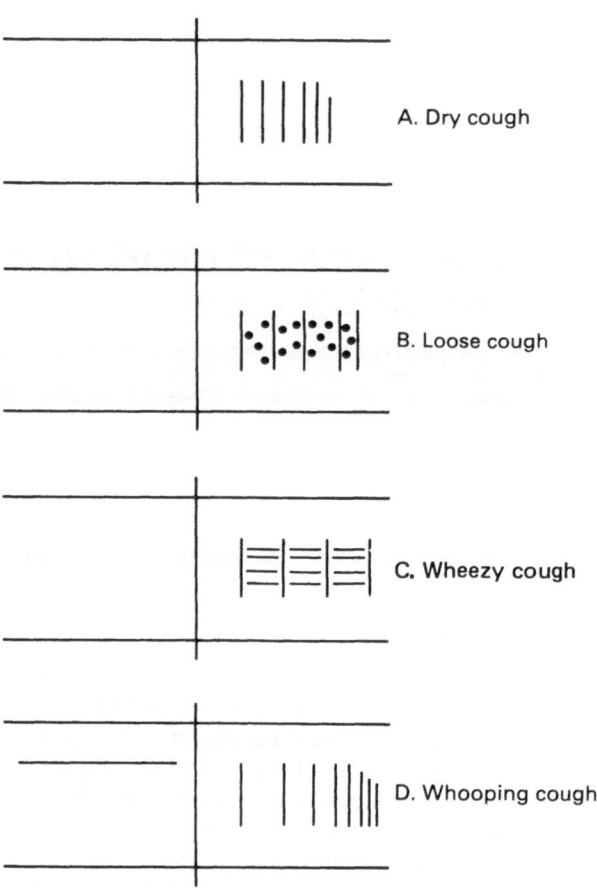

A. Dry cough

B. Loose cough

C. Wheezy cough

D. Whooping cough

Figure 1.1

Cough (Symbols explained in Figure 1.6)

sounds (Figure 1.1A). In some patients these interrupted breath sounds are replaced by a rattle, which determines the distinctive character of a loose cough (Figure 1.1B). In others a wheeze bridges successive closures of the glottis (Figure 1.1C). Both the loose and the wheezy cough are common signs of bronchitis.

Inspiratory stridor and the accelerating rhythm of coughing are well known signs of pertussis (Figure 1.1D). The term 'croupy cough' is sometimes used when the glottic sounds are faint and ill defined. Like a hoarse voice with which it is often associated, a croupy cough is a sign of laryngeal disease.

When laryngeal paralysis interferes with closure of the glottis, an interrupted low-pitched musical note, described as bovine cough replaces the explosive sounds.

Cough syncope

A severe bout of coughing may end in loss of consciousness. Cough syncope is a variety of postural fainting. The transient rise of blood pressure during a fit of coughing causes reflex peripheral vasodilatation. This leads to a sudden fall of blood pressure when the coughing ends and the intrathoracic pressure returns to normal. Patients may be reassured that these alarming episodes do not endanger life, but in order to avoid injury they should sit down during severe bouts of coughing.

Sputum

The small volume of mucus secreted by normal bronchi is swept out by the cilia and is swallowed unconsciously together with saliva and mucus from the upper respiratory tract. The earliest manifestation of chronic bronchitis is an increase of bronchial mucus which accumulates in the airways and is coughed up.

Colour

Uninfected sputum is transparent, white or grey. Infected sputum contains pus which may be evenly distributed, or form small yellow flakes suspended in mucus. The rule that yellow sputum is a sign of infection is generally valid, except in some cases of asthma where large numbers of eosinophils may form yellow plugs. At first sight these may be mistaken for pus, but eosinophils can be readily distinguished from pus cells under the microscope.

Smell

Fresh sputum is odourless. Foul smell is produced by anaerobic organisms and suggests bronchiectasis, lung abscess or a bronchopleural fistula communicating with an empyema.

Viscosity

The viscosity of sputum can be roughly estimated by pouring it from one pot into another. Recognition of viscid sputum is important in the management of asthma and of dehydration in acute respiratory infections. Occasionally the sputum contains small yellow cylindrical casts of the bronchi, consisting of inspissated mucus mixed with desquamated cells, eosinophils and fungus mycelia. These plugs are a characteristic feature of allergic bronchopulmonary aspergillosis.

Volume

The volume of sputum seldom exceeds 50 ml in 24 hours. Large amounts of purulent sputum suggest infection of a bronchiectatic lobe, lung abscess or a bronchopleural fistula com-

13

municating with an empyema or a subphrenic abscess. Profuse colourless sputum, in excess of 200 ml (bronchorrhoea) is an occasional symptom of alveolar cell carcinoma. It also occurs as a rare disease of unknown aetiology which may respond to treatment with corticosteroids.

Haemoptysis

Bleeding from the nose or gums may be reported as haemoptysis. There is occasionally some doubt as to whether the blood was coughed up or vomited. But most patients give a sufficiently clear account of the incident to diagnose bleeding from the lung on the history alone.

The implications of blood-stained sputum and a frank haemoptysis are different. The source of pure blood suddenly filling the mouth is a major blood vessel, while blood mixed with mucus or pus usually originates from the alveolar or bronchial capillaries.

Blood-stained sputum

Acute respiratory infections
The most common source of blood-stained sputum is capillary bleeding from the inflamed bronchial mucosa in acute infections complicating chronic bronchitis. An important point in the history is the change of colour from transparent mucus to yellow pus before the sputum becomes blood-streaked.

Infarct
Uniformly bloody sputum, preceded by chest pain but without symptoms of an infection, should raise the suspicion of pulmonary infarction.

Cancer
In patients who are in apparently good health blood-stained sputum may be the first sign of a small ulcerated intrabronchial tumour.

X-ray
The chest X-ray is often normal, but it may show lobar or segmental consolidation. Whether this is interpreted as pneumonia, infarction or obstruction by a tumour depends on the associated clinical features. In the absence of symptoms of an acute respiratory illness the discovery of an airless lobe is strong presumptive evidence of cancer.

Sputum tests
The sputum should be examined for neoplastic cells as soon as the bleeding has stopped. A culture for tubercle bacilli is also desirable, although tuberculosis with a normal chest X-ray is unlikely. The sedimentation rate, a traditional test for tuberculosis, is of no diagnostic value.

Bronchoscopy
Bronchoscopy will occasionally reveal a silent intrabron-

14

chial tumour, but in most cases appearances are normal. Immediate bronchoscopy is not indicated unless the previous history or the X-ray suggest that cancer is probable. An intrabronchial tumour that has bled once is likely to bleed again. Recurrence of even minimal staining of the sputum should be regarded as an immediate indication for bronchoscopy.

For those who remain in good health and present no further symptoms of pulmonary disease, a second X-ray 4 weeks later is sufficient. If this is again normal they may be dismissed from observation.

Frank haemoptysis

Mitral stenosis

The source of a sudden pulmonary haemorrhage is seldom revealed by clinical signs at the first examination. The heart should always be carefully examined for signs of mitral stenosis before the bleeding is attributed to pulmonary disease.

Bronchiectasis

Unsuspected lobar fibrosis and bronchiectasis may be discovered by a chest X-ray after a haemoptysis in patients who cannot recall any previous respiratory illness. The damage is usually the result of a forgotten episode of suppurative pneumonia or unrecognized primary tuberculosis in childhood.

Bronchiectasis confined to a single lobe is an uncommon source of haemoptysis because these destructive infections are now prevented or effectively treated. The term 'middle lobe syndrome' was applied in the past to accidentally discovered fibrosis of the middle lobe, damaged by primary tuberculosis in childhood and presenting with haemoptysis in adults. Like other late complications of primary tuberculosis it is now mainly of historical interest.

Tuberculosis

When undiagnosed tuberculosis was still common, the X-ray often revealed an unsuspected cavity as the source of a large haemoptysis. Today it is unusual to find such advanced disease, except in immigrant communities.

Aspergillus mycetoma

A previously uncommon cause of haemoptysis has taken the place of bleeding from tuberculous cavities. The source of the haemorrhage is a healed cavity, colonized by *Aspergillus fumigatus*. The X-ray may show this mycetoma as a spherical mass in the cavity. The diagnosis is confirmed by the demonstration of precipitating antibodies to *Aspergillus* in the serum.

Management

The amount of blood lost during a pulmonary haemorrhage is seldom large enough to threaten life. Death is due to asphyxia

15

from flooding of the central bronchi. The objective of emergency treatment is to keep the airways open.

The foot of the bed should be raised and the patient turned on the side of the bleeding, if this can be recognized by clinical signs. Facilities for intubation, suction and the administration of oxygen should be available. Sedation to allay anxiety is permissible, but only if ventilation is adequate. Other drugs aimed at control of the bleeding are ineffective, and insertion of a bronchial block is seldom possible. In continued or recurrent severe haemoptysis thoracotomy and ligation of the bleeding vessel should be considered as a last resort.

Dyspnoea

Breathlessness during strenuous exertion is a familiar experience in normal health. Exercise tolerance in anaemia or convalescence from a severe illness is limited by a similar discomfort. The dyspnoea in most respiratory and cardiovascular diseases is entirely different. Its precise description is beyond the verbal resources of most patients, but tightness, pressure, suffocation and inability to expand the chest indicate the wide range of distressing sensations experienced in pathological breathlessness.

Physiology   An elaborate sensory network carries information to the central nervous system about the tension exerted by the respiratory muscles, the resulting volume changes in the thoracic cage and the pressures inside the chest. Conflicting information received from these sources results in awareness of the normally unconscious act of breathing. Dyspnoea usually reflects the abnormal effort of drawing air through obstructed airways or into poorly distensible lungs. Chemical stimuli by excess carbon dioxide and hypoxia play only a secondary role.

Breathing patterns   The rate and depth of breathing, both in health and disease, is regulated in order to achieve the most economical pattern in terms of respiratory work. The work of breathing against a high expiratory flow resistance can be minimized by keeping the expiratory pressure low. Patients with airflow obstruction therefore adopt a pattern of slow expiration with short inspiration (Figure 1.2a). When the lung is poorly distensible, as in fibrosing alveolitis or interstitial pulmonary oedema, respirations are shallow and rapid (Figure 1.2b).

Chronic bronchitis   Dyspnoea in chronic bronchitis is due to the increased effort of expiration through narrowed airways. Many patients learn to live within the limits of their exercise tolerance and do

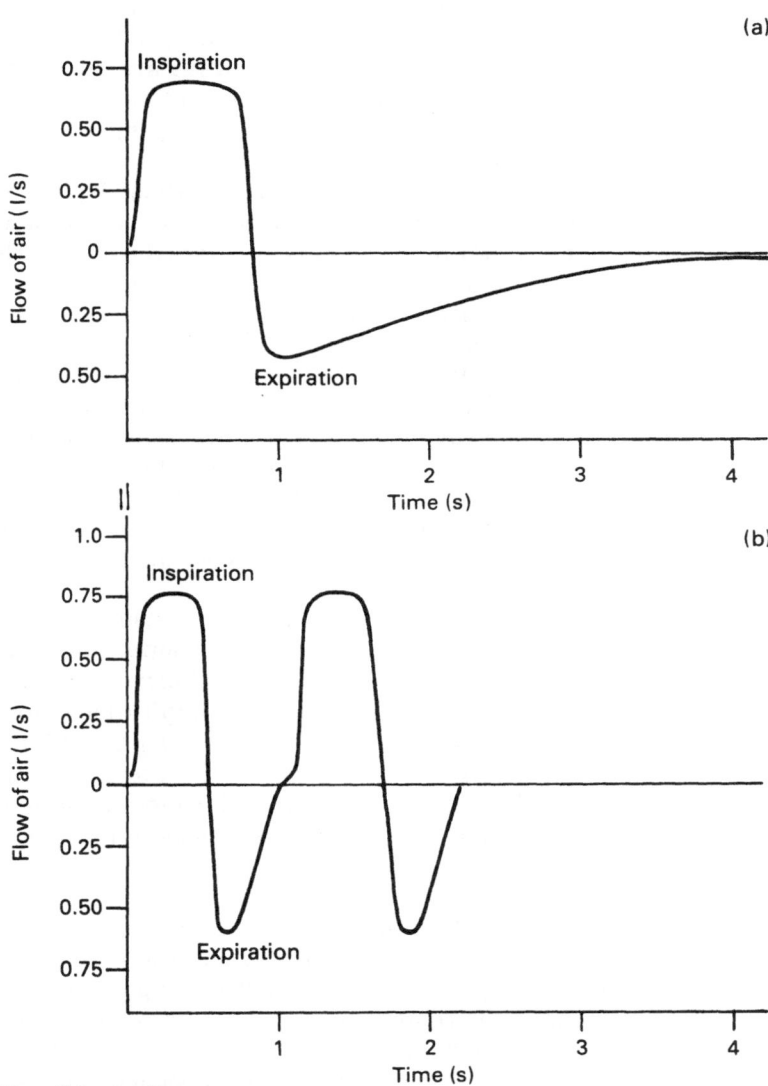

Breathing patterns
a   Widespread airflow obstruction
b   Fibrosing alveolitis

Figure 1.2

not complain of breathlessness until their peak expiratory flow rate is far below the predicted normal value. Because of this tolerance the onset of exertional dyspnoea after an acute respiratory infection may appear to be sudden.

The dyspnoea is associated with tightness over the ster-

17

num and upper ribs. Unlike angina pectoris this sensation is not painful and does not radiate outside the chest. It is at its worst on rising, when the airways are obstructed by sputum accumulated during the night, and eases gradually over the next few hours. Breathlessness on going out of doors, or while undressing in a cold bedroom, is probably due to reflex increase of the depth of respiration. Nocturnal attacks of dyspnoea are uncommon. Urgency or incontinence of micturition is often reported during severe dyspnoea. The mechanism of this distressing symptom is not known.

Asthma

Dyspnoea in asthma, as in chronic bronchitis, is due to widespread narrowing of the airways. In order to increase the calibre of the airways these patients adopt an inspiratory posture during attacks. The effort required to maintain the chest in a hyperinflated posture is an additional source of respiratory distress. It is responsible for the difficulty of getting air into the chest, aggravating the sense of expiratory obstruction. The dyspnoea is associated with tightness in the chest, varying from a mild discomfort to the acute distress of impending suffocation.

Emphysema

In primary emphysema breathlessness on exertion results from premature closure of poorly supported airways. Inspiration is not impeded, so that the pattern of breathing adopted by these patients is a slow laboured expiration followed by a short rapid inspiratory gasp. They often hyperventilate, for reasons that are not fully understood. The cause of disproportionately severe dyspnoea and hyperventilation with scanty clinical signs may not be recognized until lung function tests reveal gross abnormalities of expiratory flow rate and gas transfer.

Pulmonary embolism

Severe breathlessness and hyperventilation of sudden onset are common presenting symptoms of pulmonary embolism. When they are associated with chest pain and haemoptysis the diagnosis is relatively easy. In the absence of these symptoms of pulmonary infarction the vascular occlusion may be missed.

It is even more difficult to recognize pulmonary embolism when the pulmonary vascular bed is gradually occluded by a succession of small emboli over a long period. There is increasing dyspnoea and hyperventilation, often without other clinical signs. Evidence of pulmonary hypertension and heart failure appears late in this disease.

Spontaneous pneumo- thorax

Another cause of sudden dyspnoea and chest pain is spontaneous pneumothorax. The pain ceases within a day or two and the breathlessness rapidly improves as the lung re-

18

expands. Unilateral absence of breath sounds with a resonant percussion note are characteristic diagnostic signs.

Pulmonary oedema In pulmonary oedema the water content of the lungs is increased. At first the excess water is confined to connective tissue, particularly the sheaths surrounding the basal vessels and bronchi. This results in narrowing of the airways and impaired distensibility of the lung. The airways and alveoli are flooded later, when the lymphatic drainage of the lung can no longer cope with the amount of oedema fluid escaping from the pulmonary capillaries.

Paroxysmal dyspnoea in interstitial pulmonary oedema may be mistaken for bronchial asthma. Wheezing is common in both conditions. But the breathing pattern in pulmonary oedema, unlike that in airflow obstruction, is shallow and rapid, reflecting the impaired distensibility of the lung. Another important distinctive feature is orthopnoea. Patients with airflow obstruction often prefer to sit up in order to bring their accessory muscles into play, but they can lie flat. In pulmonary oedema the increase of intrathoracic blood volume on lying down provokes immediate distress and a rise in the rate of respiration.

Flooding of the airways by massive transudation of oedema fluid is accompanied by intense dyspnoea, akin to drowning. Only a torrential haemoptysis or sudden evacuation of a large collection of pus produces comparable acute distress.

Fibrosing alveolitis Other diseases characterized by impaired distensibility of the lung (e.g. fibrosing alveolitis) are also associated with dyspnoea and rapid, shallow breathing on exertion. This is often accompanied by an unproductive cough and retrosternal tightness or pain. In contrast to pulmonary oedema there is no orthopnoea.

Anaemia Breathlessness in anaemia, with increased rate and depth of respiration, is similar to that associated with strenuous effort in healthy subjects, except that it is provoked by inappropriately light exertion.

Effort syndrome Many other patients convalescing from an acute illness or an operation complain of impaired exercise tolerance. It also occurs among apparently healthy subjects of sedentary habits, when called upon to undertake unaccustomed exercise, for example in military training. Undue breathlessness with tachycardia, sweating, faintness and retrosternal discomfort was a common problem in wartime. This 'effort syndrome' also occurs in civilians, especially during periods of depression and emotional stress.

19

Compulsive sighing   An unfamiliar but not uncommon variety of breathlessness, also associated with depression is compulsive sighing. These patients complain from time to time of a sensation of pressure or constriction over the lower ribs, creating the illusion of restricted chest expansion and insufficient air intake. Each inspiration seems to fall further short of its target, until the desire to take a deep breath can no longer be resisted. A single maximal inspiration or a yawn gives immediate relief, but the discomfort soon returns, culminating within a minute or two in another deep inspiration.

This cyclical respiratory discomfort recurs at unpredictable intervals, day after day, over several months, usually at rest in a relaxed posture, particularly when the patient is tired. The spirogram shows an even sequence of normal tidal volumes, interrupted at regular intervals by a single deep inspiration to full vital capacity (Figure 1.3).

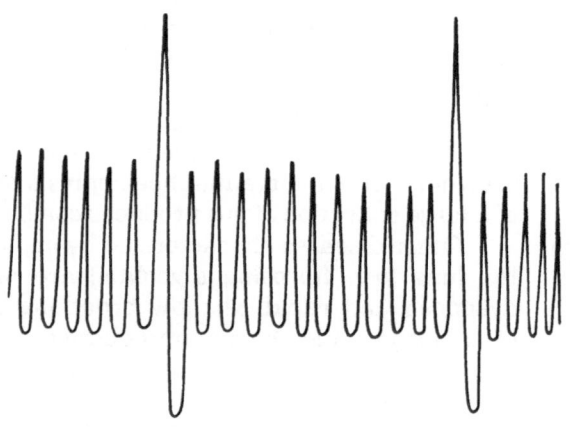

Spirogram in compulsive sighing

Figure 1.3

There is usually no sign of respiratory disease and the lung function tests are normal, except for an abnormally short breath holding time of less than 30 seconds. This complaint is often regarded as a psychoneurotic symptom and is included among other respiratory manifestations of emotional stress. Some of its features, for example the cyclical pattern, suggest that compulsive sighing may be a disorder of the central control of respiration.

Laryngeal spasm   Nocturnal attacks of sudden intense dyspnoea, due to laryngeal spasm, are liable to be mistaken for asthma if details of the history are overlooked. Characteristic features are a feeling of almost complete respiratory obstruction with stridor, lasting for less than a minute, followed by sudden relief. These episodes of paroxysmal nocturnal dyspnoea tend to recur over several years with long intervals of normal health. The circumstances of the attacks suggest that the laryngeal spasm is often provoked by regurgitation of acid gastric contents in patients with gastro-oesophageal reflux.

Pain

The lung has a rich supply of autonomic nerves. Their function is to regulate the calibre of the airways, vary the pattern of breathing and trigger the cough reflex. With the exception of retrosternal discomfort in tracheitis, stimuli applied to the lung are painless. Chest pain associated with pulmonary diseases arises from the parietal pleura or the chest wall.

Acute chest pain

Pleurisy Inflammation of the parietal pleura in pneumonia, pulmonary infarction and tuberculous pleurisy is accompanied by unilateral chest pain. Its intensity varies from a mild diffuse ache provoked by coughing to a sharply localized stabbing pain of excruciating severity which makes deep breathing or coughing intolerable. Severe pleural pain referred to the abdomen for the 8th to 10th thoracic segments may be mistaken for an acute abdominal emergency. Similarly the pain of diaphragmatic pleurisy, referred to the shoulder and neck, may be attributed to arthritis or cervical spondylosis. The diagnosis of acute pleurisy may be confirmed by a pleural rub, an effusion, or the associated symptoms and signs of pulmonary consolidation.

Spontaneous pneumo- thorax The onset of spontaneous pneumothorax is usually accompanied by unilateral chest pain. This disappears within a day or two, long before the air is completely absorbed. It is presumably a variety of pleural pain, though its mode of origin is not fully understood. A confident clinical diagnosis is possible when the breath sounds are absent over a hemithorax resonant to percussion. A small pneumothorax confined to the apex cannot be demonstrated by clinical signs and may be detected only by a chest X-ray.

Fractured rib Chest pain aggravated by deep breathing and coughing is often described as pleural, although the characteristics of pain

21

arising from other structures of the chest wall are identical. A common problem in clinical practice is whether a sharply localized pain of sudden onset is due to pleurisy or to a fractured rib. The diagnosis is relatively easy when the pain follows an injury and there are no associated respiratory symptoms. It may be very difficult when a cough fracture is a complication of chronic bronchitis or asthma. Inhibition of the cough by pain may then lead to sputum retention followed by atelectasis and infection. If the fracture is invisible on the chest X-ray the diagnosis may remain in doubt until a callus is revealed several weeks later.

Root pain Acute chest pain referred from the thoracic spine presents no difficulty when it is bilateral or is accompanied by other signs of a spinal lesion. Apart from obvious injuries, the most common cause of acute thoracic root pains is collapse of a vertebra, undermined by an unsuspected metastatic tumour.

Shingles Severe unilateral chest pain referred along one of the thoracic roots may be the presenting symptom of herpes zoster. The diagnosis may be suspected from the strictly segmental localization of the pain, and confirmed when the characteristic rash appears a few days later.

Chronic chest pain

Tuberculous pleurisy A characteristic symptom of primary tuberculous pleurisy is recurrent mild chest pain, weeks or months before the effusion appears. These episodes are often mistaken for rheumatism or intercostal neuralgia. They are presumably due to repeated minor infections of the pleura from an adjoining reservoir of tuberculous pus. (p. 124)

Cancer of the lung Recurrent chest pain is common in cancer of the lung. It is usually a symptom of pleurisy, secondary to infection in the occluded territory of the lung and may respond to treatment with antibiotics.

Carcinomatosis of the pleura is usually painless. Large effusions often accumulate silently and are not discovered until they cause breathlessness.

Severe chest pain in cancer of the lung suggests a spinal metastasis or rib erosion. An apical tumour infiltrating the upper ribs and the brachial plexus usually presents with persistent aching in the shoulder, extending into the arm.

Mesothelioma Mesothelioma, a tumour of the pleura, is often due to exposure to asbestos dust many years earlier. Persistent chest pain is a common presenting symptom at a stage when radiological appearances are still ambiguous. Advancing infiltration of the chest wall is accompanied by increasing severe, intractable pain.

Costochon-
dritis
Chondritis of one of the upper four costal cartilages (Tietze's disease) is associated with chronic or recurrent pain. The affected cartilage is tender and swollen. This is an uncommon cause of chest pain in a benign self-limiting condition of unknown aetiology.

CLINICAL SIGNS

Percussion – Auscultation: breath sounds, wheezes, crackles, pleural sounds – Clubbing of the fingers – Cyanosis – Pursed-lip breathing

Percussion

Gross structural changes in the lungs and pleura are easily detected by percussion, but the accuracy of this relatively crude test should not be overestimated. The difference between stony and lesser degrees of dullness is seldom sufficiently clear to distinguish consolidation from an effusion. The distinction between a normally resonant and hyper-resonant percussion note is also of doubtful clinical significance. Obliteration of the hepatic and cardiac dullness is common in all varieties of widespread airflow obstruction. It is due to the inflated posture of the chest and is not a specific sign of emphysema. If a chest X-ray is available, percussion is superfluous, because any condition associated with an abnormal percussion note will be visible on the film.

Auscultation
Breath sounds

Noisy
breathing
One of the best signs of airflow obstruction is noisy breathing. The breath sounds of a healthy subject are inaudible at a distance. Many chronic bronchitics and asthmatics breathe so noisily that their respirations can be heard as soon as they enter the consulting room. The noise is intensified by bronchoconstriction and reduced by bronchodilator drugs (Figure 1.4). Its loudness correlates well with the forced expiratory volume in one second (FEV_1) and the peak expiratory flow rate (PEFR) (Figure 1.5).

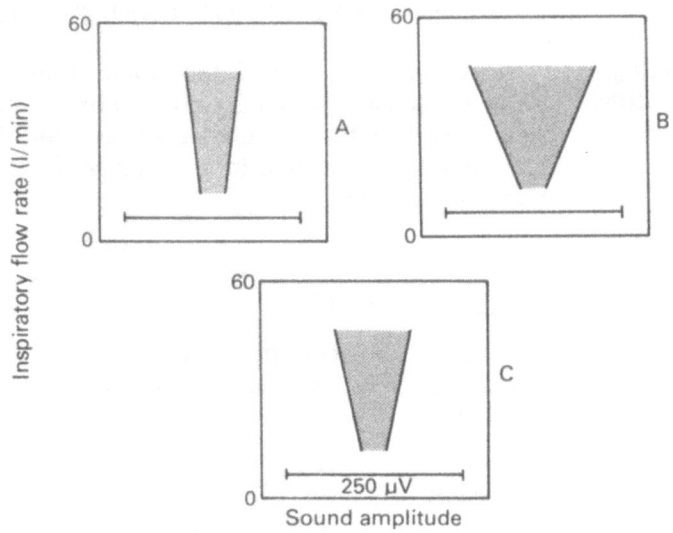

Amplitude of inspiratory breath sounds at the mouth
The increase in the amplitude of the breath sounds with rising inspiratory flow rate is greater in chronic bronchitics than in normal subjects. The noise is reduced after inhalation of a bronchodilator aerosol
A   Normal
B   Chronic bronchitis
C   Chronic bronchitis after bronchodilator aerosol

Figure 1.4

Bronchial
stenosis

There are two exceptions to this correlation. One is focal narrowing of the trachea or a large bronchus, due to tumour, foreign body, or scarring, where the noise generated at the stenosis is much louder than predicted from the FEV_1. These focally generated breath sounds can also be identified by their higher pitch and the fact that in stenosis of a lobar or segmental bronchus they are out of phase with the respiratory cycle.

Emphysema

The other exception is primary emphysema, where the inspiratory breath sounds are faint or inaudible, even when the FEV_1 and PEFR indicate severe expiratory obstruction. This is a valuable clinical sign in a disease that cannot be easily distinguished at the bedside from other varieties of widespread airflow obstruction (Figure 1.5).

Transmission
of breath
sounds

Sounds generated in the upper air passages, trachea and central bronchi are attenuated and filtered in transmission through the chest. The loudness of the inspiratory breath sounds heard through the chest wall depends partly on the gas

24

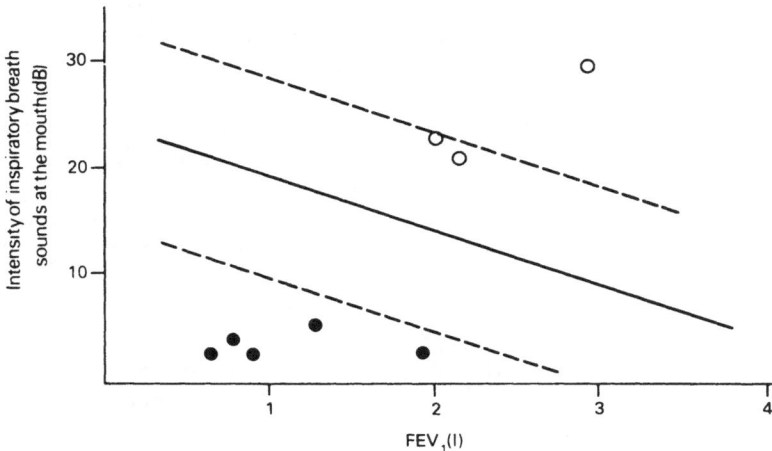

Figure 1.5

Correlation line and 95% confidence limits (dashed) between FEV_1 and intensity of inspiratory breath sounds at the mouth in chronic bronchitis. ● =primary emphysema, ○=bronchial stenosis

flow rate into the underlying territory of the lung and partly on absorption of a variable proportion of the sound by the lung and chest wall. Weak breath sounds may therefore mean impaired ventilation or poor sound transmission, and should not be interpreted as a sign of poor air entry.

The breath and voice sounds transmitted through the lung are reflected and silenced by fluid or air in the pleural cavity. A thin layer of fluid selectively transmits the higher frequencies. This accounts for the high-pitched bleating quality of the voice sounds, known as aegophony, near the upper boundary of a pleural effusion. Unfiltered transmission of breath and voice sounds through solid lung is responsible for the triad of classical signs of consolidation: bronchial breathing, bronchophony and whispering pectoriloquy.

Wheezes (rhonchi)

Wheezes are musical lung sounds. They may be audible at a distance or only through the chest wall. This depends on their loudness, so that the customary distinction between wheezing and rhonchi is superfluous. Wheezing is generally regarded as a sign of narrowing of the airways, although a simple reduction of bronchial calibre produces only noisy breathing. Musical sounds are not generated until the opposite walls of the bronchus come into contact and oscillate like the reed of a wind instrument. Wheezing is a sign of extreme bronchial narrowing, just short of complete occlusion.

Pitch

Another misconception is that high and low pitched wheezes arise from small and large bronchi respectively. This is the basis of the widespread notion that high pitched wheezing is a sign of peripheral bronchial spasm. In fact wheezes of high or low pitch can be generated anywhere in the bronchial tree, depending on the mass and elastic properties of the tissues set into oscillation.

Monophonic wheezes

Wheezing characterized by individual musical notes of well defined pitch is a common sign of chronic bronchitis and asthma. It indicates extreme narrowing of a bronchus by swelling of the mucosa or spasm. These monophonic wheezes may be inspiratory, expiratory, single or multiple, following one another at unpredictable intervals (Figure 1.6). Their number is never large because light closure of a bronchus, just short of occlusion, is uncommon. The illusion of innumerable wheezes in asthma is due to their wide transmission. The same cluster of sounds is heard with different relative loudness wherever the stethoscope is applied to the chest wall.

Figures 1.6 – 1.10

In these diagrams wheezes are represented by horizontal lines and crackles by dots. The position of these symbols on the stave corresponds to their pitch. The distance from the vertical line dividing inspiration from expiration indicates their timing

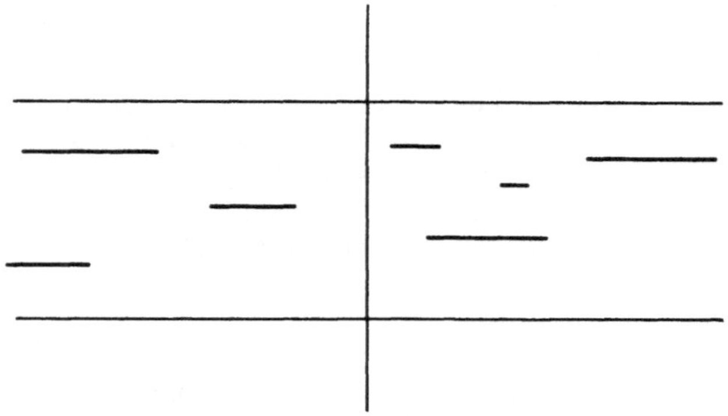

Random sequence of monophonic wheezes in asthma

Figure 1.6

Bronchial stenosis due to tumour, foreign body or scarring may be accompanied by a single persistent low pitched wheeze (Figure 1.7). This sound often remains constant for several

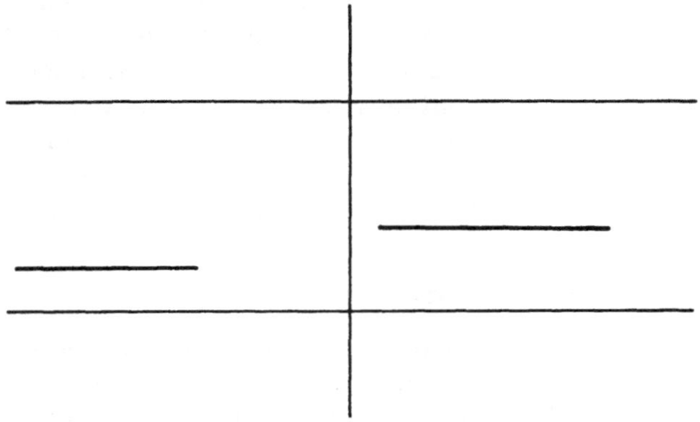

Low pitched monophonic wheeze in carcinoma of a main bronchus

Figure 1.7

days but may be silenced temporarily by a change of posture.

Stridor

Stridor is a loud low pitched musical sound, audible at a distance. Like other monophonic musical sounds it is a sign of extreme narrowing of an airway, just short of occlusion. The exceptional loudness of stridor, compared with wheezing, indicates that its source is near the mouth, usually at the larynx or in the trachea.

Polyphonic wheeze

The most common variety of wheezing is a complex musical sound confined to expiration, heard at the mouth as well as through the chest. It contains several notes of different pitch, starting and ending simultaneously, like a dissonant chord (Figure 1.8). In this respect it differs from multiple monophonic wheezes, which start and end at random intervals.

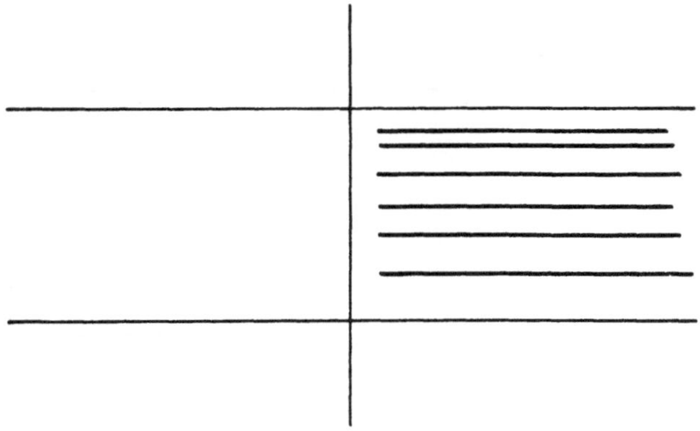

Expiratory polyphonic wheeze in widespread airflow obstruction

Figure 1.8

27

This expiratory polyphonic wheeze is a sign of simultaneous compression of several central bronchi. (p. 32) and Fig. 1.11 (p. 31). It can be produced at will by healthy subjects, but only during a violent expiration. In patients with widespread airflow obstruction it accompanies resting or mildly forced expiration. It is one of the most constant auscultatory signs of chronic bronchitis, asthma and emphysema.

Crackles (râles, crepitations)

Crackles are short sounds, lasting less than 5 milliseconds, heard in rapid succession at the mouth or through the chest wall. The ear cannot distinguish musical from non-musical sounds in such short samples; only a rough judgement of pitch is possible.

Source   The usual explanation of bubbling in the airways applies only to patients whose central bronchi are flooded by secretions. This cannot account for crackling in conditions in which there is no sputum and where these sounds are confined to inspiration or expiration. A more plausible hypothesis is that crackles are miniature explosions generated by sudden equalization of gas pressure. This occurs when a barrier between two compartments of the lung containing gas at widely different pressures is suddenly removed.

Late expirat-   The clinical interpretation of crackles depends on their
ory crackles   timing, pitch and rhythm. One variety, indicating widespread airflow obstruction, is heard over the lower lobes towards the

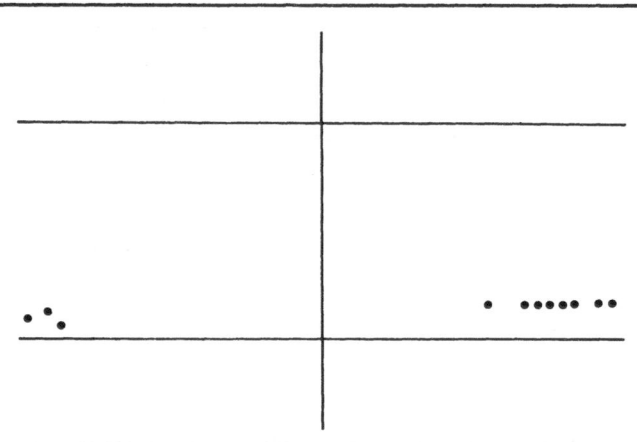

Early inspiratory and late expiratory crackles in chronic bronchitis

Figure 1.9

end of expiration and often at the start of inspiration as well. It consists of a few loud, low pitched explosive sounds, some of which may be evenly spaced (Figure 1.9). They are audible with the unaided ear or through the stethoscope held near the patient's mouth, and are not affected by changes of posture.

These crackles are produced by the passage of boluses of gas through a loosely closed large bronchus which opens intermittently whenever the upstream gas pressure is sufficient to separate its walls. Late expiratory crackling is a common sign of chronic bronchitis. It is often misinterpreted as evidence of heart failure, although the characteristics of crackling in pulmonary oedema are quite different.

Late inspiratory crackles

Crackling heard over the base of the lung in interstitial pulmonary oedema and in fibrosing alveolitis is confined to inspiration. The crackles are faint, high pitched and become more profuse towards the end of inspiration (Figure 1.10). Their spacing is at random, though the same rhythm usually recurs in several consecutive respiratory cycles. They are not transmitted to the mouth and are often silenced when the patient bends forward or lies down.

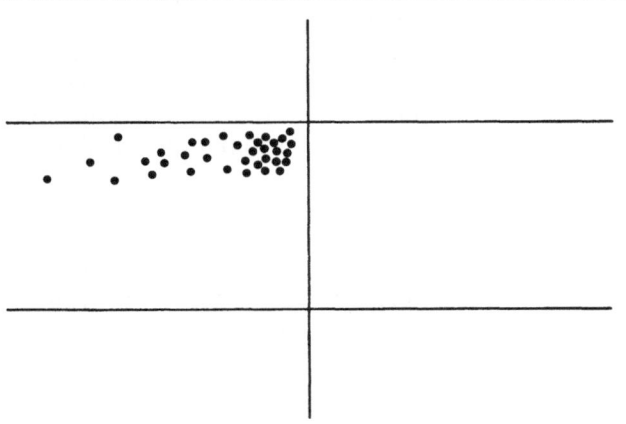

Late inspiratory crackles in fibrosing alveolitis

Figure 1.10

These explosive sounds are produced by the delayed sequential opening of peripheral basal airways. The underlying pathology is narrowing and stiffening of airways surrounded by consolidated alveoli, fibrosis, or peribronchial oedema. The upper boundary of crackling lies along a horizontal line which recedes towards the costal margin during recovery.

Pleural sounds

Pleural friction produces a series of long non-musical sounds with short interruptions. Their rhythm and timing during inspiration and expiration are often mirror images of one another. Occasionally the sounds are short and frequently interrupted, indistinguishable from pulmonary crackles.

Clubbing of the fingers

'Early' clubbing Minor changes in the shape of the nails and nailbed are often described as early clubbing. The normal limits of the angle between the nail and nailbed can be defined by measurement, but in clinical practice there is frequent disagreement whether this sign is present or absent. Early clubbing is often added to the list of observations when the diagnosis is already known, and omitted when it does not fit the rest of the clinical picture.

Gross clubbing Gross clubbing, with widening of the terminal phalanges of fingers and toes and beak shaped curvature of the nails, occurs in only a few intrathoracic diseases and is therefore of considerable diagnostic value. It may be a very early sign of a malignant tumour of the lung or pleura, appearing long before bronchial obstruction, infection or bleeding. It also occurs in intrathoracic suppuration: empyema, lung abscess or infected bronchiectasis. Gross clubbing in congenital heart disease and arteriovenous aneurysm of the lung presents no diagnostic problem, because these patients are always deeply cyanosed.

Cyanosis

The colour of the skin and mucous membranes is an insensitive test of arterial oxygen saturation. Cyanosis is often missed until saturation has fallen below 80%. Conversely, a dusky complexion in patients with sluggish peripheral circulation may be mistaken for central hypoxia. No bedside test of hypoxia is completely reliable, but inspection of the tongue in a good light is better than most. When detection of hypoxia is essential for diagnosis or treatment, there is no substitute for arterial oxygen measurements.

Pursed-lip breathing

Some patients with severe obstructive chronic bronchitis or emphysema purse their lips or grunt during expiration. This is a reliable empirical sign of severe widespread airflow obstruction, although its physiological basis is obscure.

BREATHING TESTS

Most respiratory problems can be solved without recourse to physiological measurements. In others functional data are helpful; occasionally they are indispensable. Measurement of

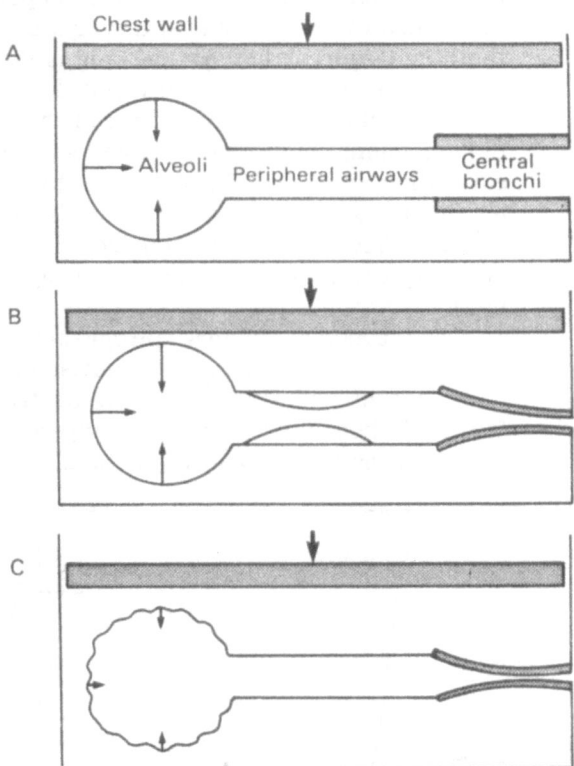

Diagram of expiratory dynamic compression of the central bronchi
A Normal. The central bronchi are kept open by the recoil pressure of the alveoli transmitted through fully patent peripheral airways
B Chronic bronchitis. The central bronchi are compressed during expiration because the recoil pressure of the alveoli is dissipated by high flow resistance in narrowed peripheral airways
C Emphysema. The central bronchi are compressed during expiration because the recoil pressure of the dilated or disrupted alveoli is abnormally low

Figure 1.11

the flow rate at the mouth during a forced expiration is essential for early diagnosis, assessment of progress and response to treatment in widespread airflow obstruction.

Expiratory flow rate
The maximum flow rate attainable during a forced expiration is limited by dynamic compression of the central bronchi, which behave like self-regulating valves. Increased effort produces a higher driving pressure, but the effect of this is cancelled by tighter compression of the bronchi. The forced expiratory flow rate over the lower two thirds or vital capacity is therefore independent of effort. It depends only on the flow resistance of the peripheral airways and the elastic recoil of the lung (Figure 1.11). As the lung is deflated the peripheral airways become more narrow and their resistance increases, while the elastic recoil pressure of the lung falls. As a result the maximum flow rate falls progressively throughout a forced expiration. In chronic bronchitis, asthma and emphysema, the maximum expiratory flow rate is abnormally low at all lung volumes. This can be demonstrated by measurement of the peak expiratory flow rate or by a spirogram recorded on a time base.

The forced expiratory spirogram is usually recorded with a portable dry spirometer. Comparison of a normal spirogram with that in widespread airflow obstruction shows the difference between the flow rates, represented by the slope of the trace and by the increased length of expiration (Figure 1.12).

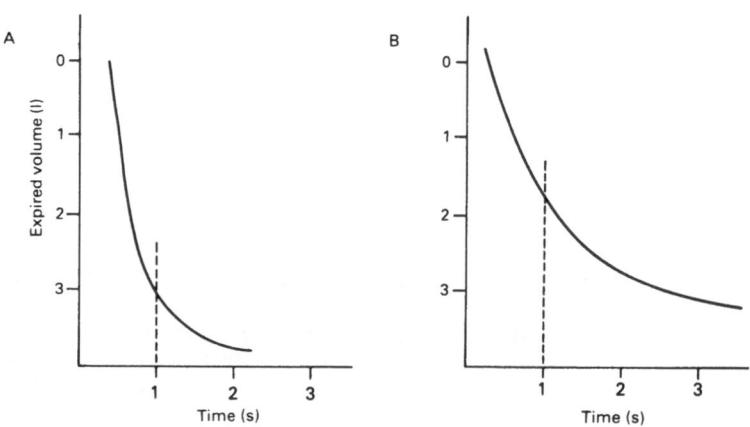

Forced expiratory spirogram
A   Normal subject
B   Widespread airflow obstruction

Figure 1.12

FEV$_1$ Among the various derivatives of the spirogram the forced expiratory volume in one second (FEV$_1$) is the measurement usually reported. It may be expressed as an absolute volume or as a percentage of the forced vital capacity (FVC). In normal subjects FEV$_1$/FVC $\times$ 100 is more than 80.

PEFR   The peak expiratory flow rate (PEFR) is recorded with an instrument which measures the flow rate at the beginning of expiration delivered with maximal force from a fully inflated chest. A short, violent puff is sufficient. False low readings can be avoided by instructing the patient to take a deep breath first and to hold the mouthpiece tightly between the lips. The Wright peak-flow meter is widely used in laboratories, but for everyday clinical work the more recently introduced peak-flow gauges are accurate enough. Normal values of PEFR are set out in Table 1.1.

Forced expiratory time   If neither a spirometer nor a peak-flow gauge is available, the forced expiratory time can be measured by timing with a stop watch the duration of the expiratory noise heard through the stethoscope over the trachea. In normal subjects it is less than 5 seconds.

Applications   Measurement of the PEFR is the most widely used test in general practice for the early diagnosis of chronic bronchitis. Abnormally low values are often recorded long before the patient complains of breathlessness. Serial measurements reflect the progress of airflow obstruction. In asthma they often give early warning of a severe attack. The effect of bronchodilator aerosols can be checked by comparison of the PEFR before, and 15 minutes after, inhalation. Response to oral bronchodilators, Intal and corticosteroids should also be checked by repeated measurements.

     Many other breathing tests are performed in departments of clinical respiratory physiology. They include studies of the gas exchange and the mechanical properties of the lung. Most common respiratory diseases can be recognized and treated without these measurements, though they often corroborate the diagnosis and provide evidence of progress.

CO transfer   One of the most useful clinical applications is measurement of the carbon monoxide transfer factor in fibrosing alveolitis. The decision whether to treat these patients with corticosteroids, and assessment of response to treatment, often depends on the trend of serial measurements. This test is also useful in the early diagnosis of asbestosis, where it may be abnormal before there is any clinical or radiological evidence of the disease.

Table 1.1 Normal values of PEFR

Women (age)	*Height* (cm)				
	150	155	160	165	170
20	410	430	440	460	480
30	390	410	420	440	460
40	360	380	400	420	440
50	340	360	380	400	420
60	320	340	360	380	400
Men (age)	*Height* (cm)				
	160	165	170	175	180
20	580	600	620	640	660
30	560	580	600	610	630
40	540	550	570	580	600
50	510	530	540	560	580
60	490	500	520	530	550

Regional function

A test widely used in the diagnosis of pulmonary vascular occlusion is external scanning of the chest after intravenous injection of a suspension of denatured serum albumin particles, labelled with a radioactive isotope. Uneven distribution of these artificial microemboli indicates defective regional perfusion, which may be due to vascular occlusion or be secondary to impaired regional ventilation. In order to distinguish these two possibilities this test is usually combined with a study of regional ventilation during inhalation of a radioactive gas.

2 Pneumonia

*Defences of the lung – Factors predisposing to infection – Class-
ification – Clinical features – Investigations – Complications –
Recurrent pneumonia – Differential diagnosis – Treatment*

Defences of the lung

The normal lung is closely guarded against bacterial infection.
Most inhaled particles are deposited in the upper respiratory
tract, others are trapped in mucus lining the bronchi, to be
swept out by the cilia. The bronchi are also protected by the
tight, closely packed arrangement of the epithelial cells, as
well as by humoral defences, including an immunoglobulin (IgA)
secreted by the submucosal plasma cells. Bacteria that may
have eluded these barriers are engulfed by alveolar
macrophages and eliminated through the lymphatic channels.

Factors predisposing to infection

Sputum
retention

Failure of these defences predisposes to acute bacterial infections. By far the most common defect is impairment of
ciliary function by excess mucus in chronic bronchitis. Sputum
retained in the airways offers a good medium for bacterial
growth. Infection is also favoured by increased viscosity and
alteration of the chemical properties of the sputum, for example in dehydration or cystic fibrosis.

35

Ineffective cough

In obstructive chronic bronchitis sputum retention is aggravated by impaired efficiency of the cough mechanism. As a result of increased flow resistance of the peripheral airways the gas flow velocity in the central bronchi is not high enough to blow sputum off the mucosal surface.

Pain

Sedatives

Debility

Cough is also ineffective when it is inhibited by pain in chest injuries and after abdominal or thoracic operations. Depression of the cough reflex by opiates and other potent sedatives contributes to the risk of postoperative pneumonia, especially in heavy smokers. Weakness of the respiratory muscles and blunting of the cough reflex is a common cause of pneumonia in many incurable diseases.

Aspiration

The lung may also become infected when its defences are overwhelmed by aspiration of septic material, such as inhaled vomit or pus from the upper respiratory tract. The source of sepsis is not always obvious, for example when small amounts of food are aspirated from a dilated oesophagus in achalasia of the cardia.

Bronchial obstruction

Structural defects

Obstruction of a major bronchus by tumour or an impacted foreign body is usually followed by infection of the occluded lobe. Less common predisposing factors are structural defects, congenital or acquired as a result of a previous infection. These include dilated or stenosed bronchi, cysts and other cavities.

Immune deficiency

Congenital immune deficiency as a cause of recurrent pneumonia is rare, but iatrogenic depression of the immune response is becoming increasingly common with the growing use of corticosteroids, immunosuppressives and cytotoxic drugs.

Viral infections

Viral infections of the respiratory tract undermine the defences of the lung and lay it open to bacterial invasion by damaging the epithelial lining of the airways. The relative role of the virus and of the secondary invader in these cases is not always clear.

Table 2.1 Pneumonia, predisposing factors

Excess sputum	Chronic bronchitis
	Bronchiectasis
Ciliary malfunction	Viscid sputum
	Dehydration
	Cystic fibrosis
Ineffective cough	Airflow obstruction
	Pain
	Debility
	Drowsiness

Pneumonia

Aspiration	Pus from URT
	Vomit
	Dilated oesophagus
Bronchial obstruction	Tumour
	Foreign body
Structural defects	Bronchial stenosis
	Cysts and cavities
Immune deficiency	Corticosteroids
	Immunosuppressives
	Cytotoxic drugs
	Congenital
Viral infections	

Classification
Bacteriological

The most logical classification of pneumonias would be bacteriological. In practice the infecting organism is seldom identified at the beginning of the illness when this would help most in the selection of antibiotics.

Bacterial infections
Bacteriological diagnosis based on the clinical features often proves to be correct. Lobar pneumonia in a previously healthy young adult is nearly always pneumococcal. Acute exacerbations of chronic bronchitis are likely to be due to *Streptococcus pneumoniae* or *Haemophilus influenzae*. Severe rapidly progressive pneumonia is often staphylococcal. In pulmonary infections secondary to bronchial obstruction, aspiration of septic material, or pulmonary infarction, a variety of bacteria, including anaerobes, are frequently involved.

Viral pneumonia
Many respiratory infections, varying in severity from a mild tracheobronchitis to fulminating pneumonia, are due to viruses. These include the respiratory syncytial virus, influenza, parainfluenza and adenoviruses. Most adults acquire partial or total immunity as a result of previous infections, so that the more severe forms of viral pneumonia occur mainly in children.

Other pathogens
Other respiratory pathogens, which may cause pneumonia clinically similar to viral infections, can be identified by serological tests. The most common amongst these is *Mycoplasma pneumoniae*. Other agents responsible for relatively rare but often severe lung infections are *Chlamydia psittaci* (psittacosis) and *Coxiella burneti* (Q fever). The most recent addition to this list is *Legionella pneumophila*, an elusive organism responsible for local outbreaks of severe pneumonia.

37

Clinical

The pathologist's definition of pneumonia is filling of the alveoli by an inflammatory exudate. This histological picture may be associated with patchy or confluent shadows on the X-ray and a wide spectrum of clinical features. These range from a trivial cough to a rapidly fatal acute illness with high fever and severe hypoxia. Between these extremes lies a large variety of clinical pictures, with or without fever, purulent sputum and airflow obstruction.

Whether such an illness is described as pneumonia, bronchopneumonia, pneumonitis, or simply as an acute respiratory infection is often a matter of opinion. The term chosen usually reflects the severity of the illness and the radiological pattern of consolidation, rather than a clear cut difference in the symptoms and signs.

The terms atypical pneumonia and pneumonitis were originally introduced to mark the difference between classical lobar and other pneumonias. They cover too many different lung infections to serve any useful purpose.

Functional

Few clinicians classify pneumonia according to its functional effects. As in other infections, the temperature, pulse rate and the level of alertness are good indications of the severity of the illness. In pneumonia the function of the lung may be profoundly affected even when these clinical signs, taken in isolation, cause no alarm. In such cases the outcome depends as much on the correct management of airflow obstruction, hypoxia and hypercapnia, as on the choice of the right antibiotic.

Clinical features
Acute bacterial infections

With the exception of pneumococcal lobar pneumonia bacterial pneumonia is usually a complication of viral infections, surgical operations, chest injuries and chronic diseases in bedridden patients. The onset is sudden, with fever, cough, purulent sputum, dyspnoea and chest pain. The textbook picture of pneumococcal lobar pneumonia is seldom seen now that antibiotics bring this illness quickly under control.

There are few differences between the presenting symptoms and signs of common bacterial pneumonias. A precise bacteriological diagnosis may be possible later from sputum cultures and response to antibiotics. The usual practice is to play safe and to start treatment with one of the wide spectrum antibiotics.

Infective exacerbations of chronic bronchitis

Increased breathlessness with relatively slight constitutional symptoms is characteristic of infective exacerbations of chronic bronchitis. In their mildest form these infections are recognized only by yellow staining of the usually white or colourless sputum. There may be slight malaise but these patients are apyrexial and do not look ill. Breathing tests show increased airflow obstruction and a diminished response to bronchodilator drugs.

The functional effects of a trivial chest infection in advanced obstructive bronchitis with chronic respiratory failure can be very serious. The arterial oxygen tension may fall dangerously low and rise of the carbon dioxide tension from an already high level leads to confusion, somnolence and coma.

Crackles at the base of the lungs are common, without clinical or radiological evidence of consolidation. The usual features of widespread airflow obstruction; restlessness, dyspnoea, noisy breathing and wheezing are often absent. The warm moist skin, strong radial pulse and normal temperature may easily create a false sense of security. Without the help of breathing tests and arterial gas measurements the seriousness of such illness is easily underestimated.

The clinical picture and hazards of chest infections are similar in chronic respiratory failure resulting from kyphoscoliosis, ankylosing spondylitis, constrictive pleurisy and after pneumonectomy.

Chronic bronchitics and other respiratory invalids are also prone to more severe acute pyrexial respiratory infections with the usual clinical features of pneumonia. Paradoxically these are often more effectively treated because the seriousness of the illness is more likely to be recognized.

Purulent sputum

Airflow obstruction

Chronic respiratory failure

Suppurative pneumonia and lung abscess

Most organisms infecting the lung do not cause tissue necrosis, so that pneumonia usually resolves completely, without cavitation or fibrosis. Primary lung infections by *Staphylococcus aureus* or *Klebsiella pneumoniae* may cause suppurative pneumonia with abscess formation.

Predisposing
factors

Apart from these specific infections a lung abscess usually means that the viability of the infected lobe has been undermined by obstruction of the draining bronchus by a tumour, inhaled septic material or infarction. The infecting organism is then of secondary importance. Cultures usually grow a mixture of several aerobic and anaerobic bacteria, not normally pathogenic in the lung.

Foul sputum
and clubbing

Persistent and profuse foul purulent sputum and clubbing of the fingers may draw attention to a lung abscess, but more often it is discovered on a chest X-ray. Further investigations include bronchoscopy, sputum cytology and culture.

Pneumonia due to viral and other non-bacterial infections

Presenting
symptoms

In contrast to bacterial pneumonias the onset of viral, mycoplasmal, chlamydial and rickettsial infections is gradual. Malaise, headache, coryza and sore throat often precede by several days the symptoms of pulmonary infection. Chest pain is common, a cough is invariably present, but the sputum may remain mucoid throughout the illness.

Progress

The clinical features of pneumonias caused by these organisms are similar, so that a precise clinical diagnosis is seldom possible. On the whole these infections are less severe than bacterial pneumonias, but they do not respond so readily to antibiotics and run a more protracted course. Clinical signs are also less clear cut. Consolidation may be demonstrable only by X-ray, though crackles and wheezes are common over the airless territories. The causal organism often remains unknown or is identified in retrospect by serological tests.

Investigations
X-rays

Patients treated at home need not be X-rayed during the acute illness if their progress is satisfactory. A chest X-ray is essential whenever response to treatment is delayed, and is advisable in all cases once the patient is ambulant.

Consolidation

Correlation between the severity of the illness and radiological appearances is not close. In non-bacterial pneumonias for example there may be extensive consolidation with relatively mild symptoms. Conversely in infective exacerbations of chronic bronchitis the patient may be on the point of death while the X-ray remains clear. The importance of radiography in the recognition of lung abscess has already been mentioned. The characteristic appearance of large ten-

Abscess

sion cavities is particularly helpful in the diagnosis of staphylococcal pneumonia.

Underlying abnormalities The main objective of a chest X-ray after recovery from pneumonia is to confirm that the consolidation has resolved. It may also demonstrate a tumour, cyst, scarring or some other unsuspected primary cause of the infection.

Sputum cultures

Interpretation of bacteriological reports on sputum presents problems which do not apply to cultures from normally sterile secretion, like urine or cerebrospinal fluid. Sputum is invari-

Contaminants ably contaminated by bacteria from the upper respiratory tract. Bacteria isolated from mucus aspirated through the

Saprophytes bronchoscope are frequently harmless saprophytes. A further source of difficulty is that some fragile pathogenic bacteria (e.g. *H. influenzae*) are easily overgrown in cultures by saprophytes, and may be missed in infections complicating chronic bronchitis.

Antibiotics In patients treated with antibiotics the cultures often represent the drug resistant survivors of a saprophytic flora, which have nothing to do with the original infection. In these circumstances it is clearly unwise to regard every organism grown from sputum uncritically as pathogenic, and even more so to change the treatment in an attempt to eradicate them. This would imply that the aim of treatment is sterilization of the sputum, an objective that is seldom attainable.

Usually pathogenic As a practical guide, a profuse growth of *Streptococcus pneumoniae* or *Staphylococcus aureus* may be accepted as evidence that these bacteria are the primary cause of the infection. *H. influenzae* and *Streptococcus pneumoniae* are the two most common pathogens in infective exacerbations of chronic bronchitis, and treatment should be designed accordingly, whether they are cultured or not.

Usually harmless Coliform bacilli and *Proteus* are often grown in profusion from the sputum of patients who have received antibiotics over a long period, and should be regarded as saprophytes. *Pseudomonas pyocyanea* is also generally harmless, but may be pathogenic, especially in cystic fibrosis and in patients with endotracheal tubes. *Klebsiella pneumoniae* is a rare cause of severe suppurative pneumonia, but like other coliform bacilli it may emerge simply as a result of intensive antibiotic treatment. Yeasts are contaminants and should be ignored, except in immune deficiencies.

41

AFB   Most laboratories culture all sputa for acid fast bacilli. Although in acute respiratory infections the result is usually negative, the occasional discovery of an unsuspected tuberculous infection justifies the labour and expense of the investigation.

Anaerobes   Repeated sputum cultures are essential when the temperature remains above normal, or purulent sputum and radiological changes persist in spite of adequate treatment with antibiotics. It is then necessary not only to exclude tuberculosis, but also to identify the organism responsible for the persistent infection. This may be an anaerobe resistant to the usual antibiotics.

Opportunist organisms   In patients whose immune defences are undermined by corticosteroids or cytotoxic drugs, an opportunist organism (e.g. *Pneumocystis carinii*, yeasts or fungi) may be responsible for the infection. In such cases it may be necessary to aspirate secretions directly from the lung, either through the bronchoscope or by transpleural needle puncture. The sample should be transferred immediately to the appropriate culture media.

Table 2.2   Sputum cultures

Probably pathogenic	*Streptococcus pneumoniae*
	Staphylococcus aureus
	Haemophilus influenzae
Probably *not* pathogenic	Coliform bacilli
	Proteus
	Pseudomonas pyocyanea
	Klebsiella pneumoniae
	Candida albicans

Sputum smears

An undeservedly neglected investigation is examination of a Gram stained sputum smear. An obvious advantage of this procedure is that the result is immediately available. Several organisms, including *Streptococcus pneumoniae*, staphyloccoci and *Klebsiella pneumoniae*, may be recognized with enough confidence to influence the choice of antibiotics.

Serological tests

These tests are helpful in the identification of non-bacterial pneumonias. A high titre of cold agglutinins or *Streptococcus* MG antibodies is a non-specific test of mycoplasmal pneu-

Cold agglutinins

42

Pneumonia

monia. It is now superseded by the more reliable complement fixation test. A rise of titre of complement fixing antibody between the first and third week of the illness is particularly significant. Unfortunately the long delay means that the result is not available when most needed as a guide to treatment.

Respiratory measurements

FEV₁ and PEFR Elaborate breathing tests are neither necessary nor feasible in patients who are too ill to co-operate. The forced expiratory volume in one second (FEV_1) or the peak expiratory flow rate (PEFR) should be measured during infective exacerbations of chronic bronchitis.

PO_2, PCO_2 In patients with severe airflow obstruction, ($FEV_1 < 1.5$ l; $PEFR < 150$ l/s) at least one arterial blood sample should be taken for measurement of oxygen and carbon dioxide tension. Hypoxia is easily missed unless cyanosis is intense. Carbon dioxide retention is clinically unrecognizable until the arterial PCO_2 is above 8 kPa (normal range 5–6 kPa). Severe hypoxia resistant to oxygen therapy and requiring urgent admission to an intensive care unit may develop with alarming speed in some viral infections.

Complications
Pleural effusion and empyema

Pleurisy The pleura is always inflamed when the infection reaches the surface of the lung. Pleurisy localized to a small area, accompanied by pain and a rub, is self-limiting and can hardly be called a complication.

Effusion When the infection spreads to a wide area of the visceral and parietal pleura, fluid accumulates in the pleural cavity and may persist long after the pneumonia has resolved.

Empyema In viral and mycoplasmal pneumonia these effusions are generally small and present no particular problem. Untreated bacterial infections may produce large purulent effusions with high fever and severe constitutional symptoms. Such effusions tend to become encysted and lead to a protracted illness with the clinical features of a chronic empyema: swinging pyrexia, high polymorph count, wasting and clubbing of the fingers.

Sterile effusions Since most acute lung infections are treated with antibiotics and their progress is checked with X-rays, chronic empyema has become uncommon. Infection of the pleura by

43

pyogenic organisms is now represented by pleural effusions sterilized by antibiotics, but persisting for some time after the pulmonary infection has resolved.

Treatment   In such cases a sample of pleural fluid should be aspirated and cultured to ascertain that it does not contain viable pyogenic organisms. If the fluid is sterile no treatment is necessary, as the fluid will be absorbed spontaneously. If the culture grows pyogenic organisms the effusion must be treated by repeated aspiration, combined with intrapleural and systemic administration of the appropriate antibiotic (p. 128). A fully developed empyema containing thick pus may also resolve under this treatment, so that surgical drainage or excision of the pleura is seldom necessary.

Fibrosis and bronchiectasis

Most lung infections resolve completely, leaving no structural or functional damage. Suppurative pneumonia complicating obstruction of a major bronchus may destroy all function in the territory beyond the obstruction, leaving dense fibrous tissue and dilated bronchi in place of the normal architecture.

Chronic suppurative pneumonia   Fibrosis and bronchiectasis confined to a single lobe was not uncommon before the introduction of antibiotics and routine removal of inhaled foreign bodies. Such a chronic suppurative pneumonia causes chronic ill health, profuse foul, purulent sputum, and clubbing of the fingers, all well described in classical texts under the heading of bronchiectasis. In others the infecting organisms die out, leaving no residual symptoms until a haemoptysis draws attention to the fibrosed lobe. This clinical picture was formerly known as dry bronchiectasis.

The prompt diagnosis of bronchial obstruction by X-ray and bronchoscopy, and effective treatment of the infection, has greatly reduced the incidence of this complication. Fibrosis and bronchiectasis confined to a single lobe, discovered by a routine X-ray or brought to light by haemoptysis or infection, is today more likely to be congenital or due to an unrecognized tuberculous infection in childhood.

Recurrent pneumonia

Chronic bronchitis   Chronic bronchitis is by far the most common cause of recurrent acute chest infections in middle age (p. 55). Such patients are often referred to clinics for an opinion as to whether they have bronchiectasis. Cylindrical dilatation of some bronchi is so common in chronic bronchitis that the relevant question is whether it contributes to the patient's ill health.

At bronchoscopy there may be as much mucus or pus in the bronchi leading to bronchographically normal territories as in bronchi with dilated peripheral branches. In others sputum in the bronchiectatic territories is more profuse than elsewhere.

In the presence of widespread bronchial disease it is unsafe to attribute recurrent pyrexial episodes with purulent sputum to infection of the most severely damaged bronchi. The results of resection in such cases are disappointing (p. 58).

Cysts and cavities Bronchiectatic lobes destroyed by suppurative pneumonia or primary tuberculosis, congenital cysts, and cavities resulting from previous infections may be secondarily infected by pyogenic organisms. Acute infections with fever and purulent sputum, accompanied by recurrent pain referred to the same part of the chest, usually draw attention to the damage in the underlying territory of the lung.

Tumour Tumours may present with recurrent infections distally to an incompletely obstructed bronchus. A small intrabronchial growth, whether benign or malignant, is not visible on the chest X-ray and the lobe supplied by the narrowed bronchus remains fully aerated until the obstruction is complete. Sputum may however be trapped at the stenosis long before then, causing intermittent atelectasis and recurrent infections.

Tuberculous bronchial stenosis The same sequence of events occurs in bronchial stenosis resulting from healed primary tuberculosis. In the past the right middle lobe was particularly vulnerable by post-tuberculous bronchial stenosis, but like other late tuberculous complications this is now very uncommon.

Aspiration pneumonia Repeated aspiration of food from the dilated oesophagus in achalasia of the cardia, and less often in gastro-oesophageal reflux, may cause recurrent pneumonia. Dysphagia and other oesophageal symptoms may not be troublesome enough to be reported. Investigation of recurrent pneumonia should therefore include a barium meal.

Immune deficiency A rare cause of recurrent pneumonia is congenital or acquired immune deficiency. It is easily recognized in patients under treatment with corticosteroids, immunosuppressives or cytotoxic drugs. In others, with hypogammaglobulinaemia and other primary immune deficiencies, detailed serological investigations are necessary.

Cystic fibrosis The most damaging complication of cystic fibrosis is recurrent infection of the lung, usually by staphylococci. These infections start in infancy and become increasingly frequent during childhood. The underlying abnormality of mucus and other exocrine secretions may not be recognized unless they are associated with intestinal symptoms. The diagnosis is confirmed by sweat sodium estimation and pancreatic function tests (p. 134).

Catarrhal children

Many young children aged 2 – 6 years are abnormally prone to recurrent short feverish illnesses with cough, wheezing, sore throat, rhinitis and earache. They are often referred to as 'catarrhal', a term which leaves the aetiology open to discussion. Certain features, especially the fever, suggest that at least some of these illnesses are viral infections. There may be other factors, including hypersensitivity to allergens. These recurrent infections usually cease long before puberty (p. 131).

Differential diagnosis
Pulmonary infarction

The differential diagnosis between pneumonia and pulmonary infarction is difficult. The presenting symptoms and signs are so similar that the two conditions may be indistinguishable at the start. Post mortem studies have shown that acute pulmonary complications in the medical and surgical wards of hospitals are often regarded as atelectasis or pneumonia when they are in fact due to occlusion, by thrombosis or embolism, of a major pulmonary artery.

Symptoms

Chest pain and breathlessness with clinical and radiological signs of consolidation are common to both conditions. Special features which should raise the suspicion of pulmonary infarction are severe dyspnoea, hyperventilation and tachycardia with a normal or slightly raised temperature, and above all, heavily blood-stained sputum in the first few hours of the illness. Confirmatory signs of right ventricular strain are often absent at this stage.

Function tests

Respiratory function tests are usually inconclusive. The results of radio-isotope tests do not distinguish pneumonia from an infarct; both ventilation and perfusion being impaired over the radiologically opaque area of the lung. Deficient perfusion in other, radiologically normal, regions of the lung is on the other hand strong supporting evidence of a vascular occlusion.

Progress

Progress during the next few days may help to clarify the diagnosis. Persistence or recurrence of heavily blood-stained sputum, further episodes of chest pain and dyspnoea, a pleural rub or consolidation in other parts of the lung increase the probability of pulmonary embolism. By then the diagnosis may be confirmed by clinical or electrocardiographic signs of right ventricular strain. Purulent sputum and pyrexia at this stage should not be regarded as evidence of a primary pneumonia, as these symptoms may be due to a secondary infection of the infarcted lung.

Tuberculous pleurisy

The presenting symptoms of tuberculous pleurisy: chest pain and pyrexia, may be mistaken for those of an acute lung infection with inflammation of the overlying pleura. Most of these patients have already received treatment with antibiotics before the diagnosis is reconsidered because of continued fever or a pleural effusion. At this stage it may be difficult to distinguish an acute pyogenic infection of the pleura, sterilized by antibiotics, from a primary tuberculous pleural effusion.

Distinctive features
An important point in the history of tuberculous pleurisy is chest pain preceding the acute illness by several weeks or months. Tuberculous effusions are also larger, persist longer, and contain a higher proportion of lymphocytes. The temperature settles more slowly, even under treatment with anti-tuberculosis drugs (p. 124).

Pulmonary tuberculosis

Tuberculous lobar pneumonia
Tuberculous pneumonia should always be considered in the differential diagnosis of an acute lung infection. Tuberculous lobar pneumonia following a primary infection is uncommon, except in infants and immigrants. Its clinical and radiological signs are identical with those of other lobar pneumonias. The diagnosis is usually first suspected when there is no response to antibiotics. The sputum always contains large numbers of acid fast bacilli.

Tuberculous broncho-pneumonia
Acute tuberculous bronchopneumonia is usually due to aspiration of sputum from a chronic tuberculous cavity. In an elderly man with a chronic cough it may be mistaken for an acute infective exacerbation of chronic bronchitis. Sputum tests and a chest X-ray are essential in these patients.

Subphrenic abscess

A subphrenic abscess masked by a pleural effusion may be mistaken for pneumonia or pleurisy if the possibility of an encysted collection of pus under the diaphragm is not considered. The clue to the diagnosis is a history of appendicitis, perforated peptic ulcer, or some other acute abdominal emergency followed by a stormy postoperative course.

The subphrenic abscess may not be recognized until continued ill health, fever and leucocytosis draw attention to a hidden collection of pus. Impaired percussion note with bronchial breathing over the lower lobe may be misinterpreted as a sign of a chest infection. The diagnosis may be difficult, even after intensive radiological investigation, and often requires exploration of the suphrenic compartments by aspiration or laparotomy.

Spontaneous pneumothorax

The presenting symptoms of spontaneous pneumothorax, sudden chest pain and dyspnoea, are similar to those of an acute lung infection with pleurisy. But there is no cough or fever, and the clinical signs, unilateral absence of breath sounds over a normally resonant chest, are characteristic. In a shallow pneumothorax, confined to the apex, a pleural rub may be the only clinical sign. This may be mistaken for pleurisy unless the chest is X-rayed.

Eosinophilic consolidation

Lobar, segmental or patchy consolidation of the lung with a high blood eosinophil count occurs in a variety of conditions, including allergic bronchopulmonary aspergillosis and hypersensitivity to drugs. It may also be the presenting illness in polyarteritis before other organs are affected. In many cases the aetiology is obscure.

Radiological appearances are similar to those of lobar or bronchopneumonia, but the temperature remains normal and the symptoms are disproportionately mild. There may be wheezing and dyspnoea; in many others the consolidation shown by the X-ray is unexpected. The clue to the diagnosis is the high blood eosinophil count, often in excess of 1000 cells/mm^3.

Carcinoma of the bronchus

An acute lung infection may be the first sign of a tumour obstructing a major bronchus. The diagnosis may be revealed by the chest X-ray or by a cytological report on the sputum, but the clinical features are indistinguishable from those of a primary pneumonia. The underlying cancer is often recognized only when the pneumonia fails to resolve or if the infection recurs.

Table 2.3 Pneumonia – differential diagnosis

Diagnosis	Distinctive features
Pulmonary infarction	Tachypnoea, heavy blood staining, deep vein thrombosis
Tuberculous pleurisy	Previous history of chest pain, persistent fever and effusion
Tuberculous pneumonia	Infants, immigrants; unrecognized chronic tuberculosis, AFB in sputum
Subphrenic abscess	Previous history of acute abdomen, swinging fever, high WCC
Spontaneous pneumothorax	Normal temperature, resonant percussion with absent breath sounds
Eosinophilic consolidation	Normal temperature, wheezing, high eosinophil count
Cancer	Delayed resolution, relapse

Treatment
Indications for admission to hospital

Pneumonia can be adequately treated at home, provided that social conditions are satisfactory. Admission to hospital is advisable for infants and the very old, also for patients at special risk, including alcoholics, diabetics and in chronic, debilitating diseases. When pneumonia is the terminal event of an incurable illness, admission to hospital is inappropriate.

All patients requiring continuous oxygen, assisted ventilation or intensive physiotherapy should be in hospital. This group includes severe bacterial or viral pneumonias. The most common indication for these special procedures is a respiratory infection in advanced chronic bronchitis. Many of these patients die at home, or soon after admission to hospital, because carbon dioxide retention is not recognized in time.

Even a relatively mild infection complicating severe chronic airflow obstruction may end in hyperkapnic coma and fatal hypoxia unless treatment is closely supervised in an intensive care unit. Respiratory infections complicating chronic respiratory failure need immediate admission, preferably by a standing arrangement with a local hospital where the patient is already known.

Antibiotics

Penicillins   Treatment with antibiotics is often started before the infecting organism has been identified. It is then advisable to choose a drug with a wide antibacterial spectrum, such as ampicillin or amoxycillin.

Pneumonia in previously healthy young adults is likely to be pneumococcal and is best treated with benzylpenicillin 600 mg (1 mega-unit) twice daily by intramuscular injection. This is inconvenient outside hospitals, and comparative studies have shown that ampicillin 250 mg, 4 times daily by mouth is equally effective.

Erythromycin
Co-trimoxazole   For patients who are hypersensitive to penicillins, erythromycin 250 mg, 4 times daily, or co-trimoxazole two tablets (each containing 80 mg trimethoprim and 400 mg sulphamethoxazole), twice daily are suitable alternatives in pneumococcal pneumonia.

Cephalosporins have no advantages over less expensive drugs. They are unsuitable for patients allergic to penicillins, because they are usually allergic to cephalosporins as well.

Flucloxacillin   In severe lung infections, especially during influenza epidemics, it is wise to choose a combination which is effective against penicillin resistant strains of *Staphylococcus aureus*. In such cases ampicillin should be supplemented by flucloxacillin 250 mg, 4 times daily by mouth. In severe pneumonia both drugs may be given by intramuscular injection during the first 48 hours.

Tetracyclines   Infective exacerbations of chronic bronchitis are usually due to *Streptococcus pneumoniae* or *H. influenzae*. The choice of antibiotic between ampicillin, oxytetracycline, co-trimoxazole and erythromycin is a matter of personal preference. None of these drugs has been shown to be clearly superior to the others. Their effect in the conventional dosage is bacteriostatic, so that the infection often recurs afer a short remission.

Longer remissions may be expected if the dose of ampicillin is increased to the bactericidal level of 1 g, four times daily during the first three days of treatment.

In lung infections attributed to non-bacterial agents oxy-

50

tetracycline is a suitable choice. Apart from their wide anti-bacterial spectrum the tetracyclines are also effective in mycoplasmal pneumonia, psittacosis and Q-fever.

Chlor-amphenicol

One of the few permissible uses of chloramphenicol is in life-threatening infections by *H. influenzae* complicating chronic respiratory failure in chronic bronchitis.

Other combinations

Other drug combinations for treatment of severe lung infections in hospital are as follows:

(1) Fusidic acid with flucloxacillin, in staphylococcal lung abscess.

(2) Gentamicin or benzylpenicillin with streptomycin, in infections due to *Klebsiella pneumoniae*.

(3) Gentamicin or metronidazole, in anaerobic infections.

(4) Carbenicillin with gentamicin, where *Pseudomonas pyocyanea* is regarded as the pathogenic organism.

Oxygen

Continuous treatment with oxygen needs close supervision in hospital. While awaiting admission it may be administered by nasal prongs at flow rates between 1 and 2 l/min, or a mask supplying low concentrations (24 – 30%) of oxygen (Ventimask, Edinburgh mask). This modest oxygen supplement is safe and sufficient in the short term to prevent fatal hypoxia. Higher concentrations of oxygen in unrecognized chronic respiratory failure may depress ventilation and lead to severe carbon dioxide retention with loss of consciousness.

Physiotherapy

The objective of physiotherapy in acute lung infections is to prevent obstruction of the airways by sputum. It is unnecessary in pneumococcal lobar pneumonia and infections by non-bacterial agents, where a sputum is scanty and easily coughed up.

Breathing exercises

Physiotherapy is an essential part of treatment in infective exacerbations of chronic bronchitis and in conditions where pain inhibits coughing. Such patients are prone to obstruction of a major bronchus by retained secretions and may develop atelectasis of the basal alveoli as a result of shallow breathing. For these reasons it is important to encourage coughing and deep breathing.

Postural
drainage
Postural drainage was an important part of treatment of lung abscess and bronchiectasis, and is still widely used. It is certainly helpful in clearing secretions from dependent territories of the lung, but since the advent of antibiotics it is no longer essential. There is no justification for subjecting elderly or breathless patients to this ordeal. The proper place of postural drainage in acute lung infections is amongst the measures used by physiotherapists to encourage coughing in a reluctant patient.

Analgesics and sedatives

Sedatives
In previously healthy young patients potent analgesics, including opiates, are permissible. In chronic bronchitis and elderly patients whose previous respiratory history is not known, analgesics must be chosen with great care and all sedatives with the possible exception of benzoctamine (Tacitin) are contraindicated. Unfortunately the risk of sputum retention is greatest in this group, leaving no alternative to vigorous and sometimes ruthless physiotherapy.

③ Chronic bronchitis

Prevalence – Pathology – Clinical features – Investigations – Differential diagnosis – Complications – Treatment

Prevalence

A perennial productive cough with recurrent chest infections is one of the most common respiratory complaints in adults.. Many, though by no means all these patients become increasingly breathless with advancing age.

Chronic bronchitis occurs all over the world, but even allowing for differences in terminology, its prevalence varies greatly between countries. It is one of the most common medical reasons for absence from work in the United Kingdom, where the mortality from the disease is also higher than in any other economically advanced country (Figure 3.1).

There is a well documented association with cold climate, air pollution, poor housing and above all, cigarette smoking. The exceptionally high mortality from chronic bronchitis in the British Isles is mainly due to smoking. Atmospheric pollution was until recently an important contributory factor.

Pathology

Mucus secretion
A widely accepted definition of chronic bronchitis is based on its earliest symptom: a productive cough, persisting for at least three months in more than two consecutive years. The cor-

53

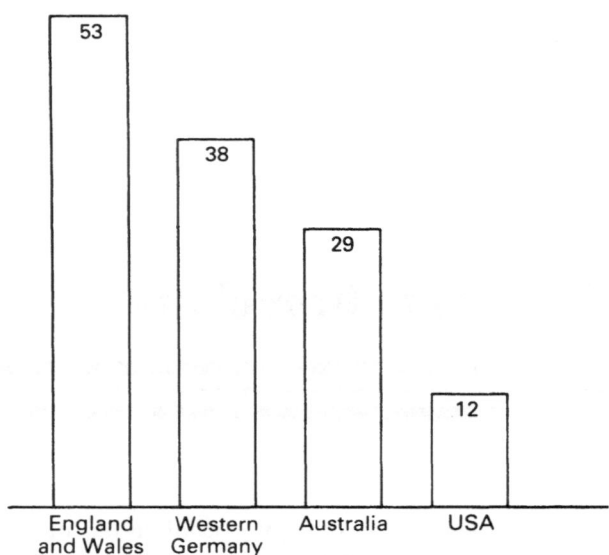

Mortality from chronic bronchitis (1975) WHO report
Death rate per 100 000 population

Figure 3.1

responding histological change is an increase in the number and size of the bronchial mucus-secreting acini.

Airflow obstruction
    Airflow obstruction begins in the peripheral airways. At this stage it does not cause breathlessness and cannot be detected by conventional breathing tests. Progressive obstruction is accompanied by increasing dyspnoea and wheezing. By then the structural changes in the walls of the larger bronchi are demonstrable as irregularities of calibre on bronchograms. Emphysema is often associated with advanced chronic bronchitis. Loss of elastic tension of the lung then contributes to limitation of the expiratory flow rate.

    Why some patients with increased bronchial mucus secretion develop airflow obstruction, while others escape, is not fully understood. Recurrent infection was thought to be the probable cause of progressive bronchial obstruction, but this hypothesis was disproved by a long-term study of the natural history of chronic bronchitis. It is possible that the airways of some subjects are abnormally vulnerable to inhaled irritants, particularly cigarette smoke. Cumulative damage, starting in childhood, may manifest itself later in life as excessive mucus secretion, or as progressive airways obstruction, or as a combination of both abnormalities.

Clinical features
Increased mucus secretion

Cough A productive cough, lasting for several weeks during the winter, is usually the first and often the only symptom of chronic bronchitis. Few patients consult their doctor at this stage, because they regard the cough as a natural and harmless result of smoking. The cough is usually worse on rising in the morning and while undressing in a cold bedroom at night. During the day it is less troublesome, unless provoked by sudden changes of temperature.

Sputum The sputum at this stage consists of bronchial mucus with an admixture of saliva. It is easily pourable, colourless, or grey when contaminated by soot. The disease may be first recognized during an acute respiratory infection or after a series of minor illnesses when the sputum becomes purulent and more profuse. After some years of recurrent winter bronchitis the cough and sputum persist throughout the year and infections with purulent sputum become increasingly frequent.

Signs The cough in chronic bronchitis has a characteristic 'loose' sound, usually attributed to the rattling of sputum in the central bronchi (p. 12). Another common clinical sign of increased mucus secretion is a series of low-pitched crackles, heard at the mouth and over the lower lobes at the beginning of inspiration and towards the end of expiration (p. 28).

Airflow obstruction

Dyspnoea Many chronic bronchitics become breathless on exertion in late middle age. At first they notice this only on stairs and hills and regard it as a natural consequence of ageing. Dyspnoea is often reported only when it begins to restrict the pace of walking on level ground.

The transition from mild to severe dyspnoea may be gradual. Often it is sudden, after an acute respiratory infection. At a more advanced stage exercise tolerance is limited to a few steps on level ground. The first hour after rising is the worst. Even washing and shaving is then a struggle, until the bronchi are cleared of sputum accumulated during the night.

Breathing pattern Breathlessness in chronic bronchitis is a symptom of widespread narrowing of the airways. As a result of increased airflow resistance in the small airways, often associated with loss of elastic tension of the lung, the central bronchi are compressed during expiration and set a limit to the flow rate (p. 32). In these circumstances prolonged slow expiration and short rapid inspiration is the most economical pattern of breathing (p. 16).

Noisy breathing A characteristic sign of widespread narrowing of the air ways is noisy breathing. The respirations of a healthy subject are inaudible at the mouth, while in obstructive chronic bronchitis they can be heard at a distance of several feet. The inspiratory noise is closely correlated with other indices of airflow obstruction and may be used as a clinical test of the severity of airway narrowing (p. 23).

Wheezing Another common sign of airflow obstruction is wheezing, particularly a polyphonic musical sound produced by the simultaneous expiratory compression of several central bronchi. This loud wheeze is transmitted to the mouth and through the chest wall. It is often audible at a distance, at rest or during a mildly forced expiration (p. 27).

Investigations

FEV₁ and PEFR Limitation of the expiratory flow rate by premature collapse of the central bronchi is demonstrable by the abnormally low

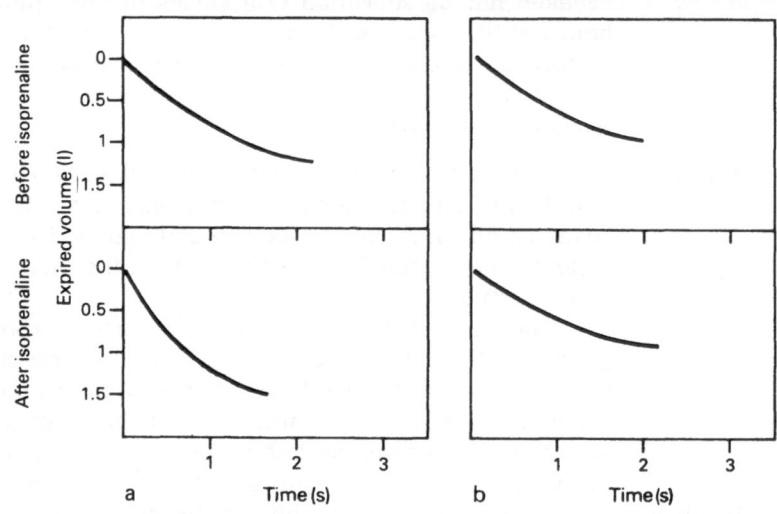

Forced expiratory spirogram in chronic bronchitis
a Reversible airflow obstruction
b Irreversible airflow obstruction
Top: before isoprenaline
Bottom: after isoprenaline

Figure 3.2

forced expiratory volume in one second (FEV_1) and peak expiratory flow rate (PEFR). Impaired performance in these tests is often the only evidence of obstructive chronic bronchitis.

Serial measurements over several years have shown that the rate of progression of airflow obstruction varies between patients. In some it is gradual, in others long periods of stability are interrupted by a sudden stepwise fall of PEFR. In favourable circumstances, especially in patients who stop smoking, the deterioration may be arrested and normal function occasionally returns.

Broncho-
dilator
response
These tests may also be used to measure the reversibility of airflow obstruction. The FEV_1 or PEFR is recorded immediately before and 5 minutes after inhalation of a single puff or isoprenaline aerosol (Medihaler Iso). Most patients respond, but in advanced chronic bronchitis with emphysema there may be no improvement (Figure 3.2).

X-ray

In the early stages of chronic bronchitis the chest X-ray is normal. In severe airflow obstruction the lungs are hyperinflated, with increase of the vertical and antero-posterior diameter of the thoracic cavity. These radiological signs do not distinguish chronic bronchitis from other causes of hyperinflation.

Occasionally the marks of a past infection such as obliteration of the costo-phrenic angle or scarring in the lung are visible. Some X-ray reports describe lungs with a rich vascular pattern as 'bronchitic', but there is no evidence that such appearances and chronic bronchitis are correlated.

Sputum tests

Cultures
If the sputum is colourless or white, there is no point in sending it for bacteriological examination. Even cultures of purulent sputum are often unrewarding. Laboratories specializing in the bacteriology of chronic bronchitis often isolate *H. influenzae* and other pathogenic organisms, but elsewhere the cultures usually grow only commensals and upper respiratory flora.

Smears
A more helpful test in acute exacerbations of chronic bronchitis is examination of a sputum smear. Some pathogenic organisms, including *Streptococcus pneumoniae*, *Staphylococcus aureus* and *H. influenzae* may be identified by their form and staining properties. Clumps of eosinophils in the sputum, especially if associated with blood eosinophilia, are a feature of allergic bronchitis.

Differential diagnosis
Tuberculosis

An enquiry into deaths from tuberculosis showed that failure to consider the possibility of this disease is still a common source of diagnostic error. A chronic cough in elderly men should not be attributed to chronic bronchitis until pulmonary tuberculosis has been excluded by a chest X-ray. If the X-ray is normal, it need not be repeated. Tuberculous scars and calcified nodules should be checked with further X-rays and sputum tests at intervals of 2–3 years. Patients under treatment with corticosteroids should be X-rayed every year.

Bronchiectasis

The bronchogram in chronic bronchitis often shows widespread abnormalities of bronchial calibre, including minor cylindrical dilatation with beading of the segmental bronchi and their branches. The clinical significance of these changes is uncertain.

When the bronchi in one lobe are much more dilated than elsewhere it may be difficult to decide whether these severely damaged bronchi are the main source of sputum and recurrent infections, or merely an incidental feature of widespread chronic bronchitis. Be that as it may, the results of resection of a bronchiectatic lobe in the presence of widespread minor calibre changes are disappointing. This is in striking contrast with the success of surgical treatment in bronchiectasis resulting from suppurative pneumonia. where the rest of the lung is healthy. In view of the poor results of surgical treatment, bronchography in chronic bronchitis is unnecessary, as the discovery of dilated bronchi is only of academic interest.

Asthma

The perennial symptoms of chronic bronchitis are different from the episodic airway obstruction of asthma. Nevertheless a persistent cough, sputum and dyspnoea starting in middle age is sometimes labelled as asthma when it is associated with eosinophilia or if it responds to treatment with corticosteroids. Differences of opinion about the diagnosis in these patients reflect the lack of consensus about the definition of asthma (p. 74).

Complications
Emphysema

Emphysema is defined as enlargement of the alveoli beyond normal anatomical limits, usually accompanied by destruction of their walls. This diagnostic label is often added to that of chronic bronchitis without any proof that the alveoli are dilated or ruptured. Emphysema is in fact often associated with chronic bronchitis, but the clinical features of these two conditions are so similar that the diagnosis is unreliable unless it is supported by radiological evidence and respiratory function tests.

Emphysema is probable when severe irreversible expiratory obstruction, indicated by a very low FEV_1 or PEFR, is associated with quiet inspiratory breath sounds at the mouth. The carbon monoxide transfer factor is reduced, but the arterial gas tensions are normal. Measurement of the total lung capacity shows that the chest in full inspiration is distended beyond physiological limits.

The chest X-ray may show bullae circumscribed by thin circular lines. In others the presence of emphysematous territories can be inferred from uneven distribution of blood vessels. Radiological signs of hyperinflation are sometimes reported as emphysema, but as they are common to all varieties of widespread airflow obstruction their diagnostic value is. unreliable.

Cor pulmonale

Equivocal signs

Cor pulmonale is another diagnostic label added to that of chronic bronchitis and emphysema on flimsy evidence. The early inspiratory basal crackles in chronic bronchitis are due to intermittent closure of a large bronchus and have nothing to do with pulmonary oedema. Distension of the neck veins reflects the high expiratory intrathoracic pressure and should not be interpreted as evidence of heart failure. Severe dyspnoea and cyanosis are common to both conditions. In these circumstances the diagnosis of heart failure is unreliable unless it is supported by oedema, triple rhythm and electrocardiographic evidence of right ventricular strain.

Pathogenesis

The association between chronic bronchitis and heart failure may be fortuitous, since coronary ischaemia and hypertension are common in elderly patients. When heart failure is the direct result of chronic bronchitis, the link between the two conditions is water retention associated with hypercapnia, or pulmonary hypertension due to hypoxia.

Hypercapnic dropsy and hypoxic pulmonary hypertension occur only in a small group of chronic bronchitics who are in respiratory failure. Measurement of arterial blood gases is therefore an essential investigation in the diagnosis of cor pulmonale complicating chronic bronchitis.

Chronic respiratory failure

Blood gases Respiratory failure is defined in terms of impaired gas exchange: a reduction of arterial PO_2 below 8 kPa (60 mmHg) or a rise of arterial PCO_2 above 6 kPa (45 mmHg). Mild hypoxia in chronic bronchitis is common by the time dyspnoea begins to limit exertion. During acute exacerbations the arterial gas tensions may be grossly abnormal, but they return to their usual value as soon as the crisis is over.

In a few patients with severe airflow obstruction the hypercapnia and severe hypoxia persist. These patients, in chronic respiratory failure, are at special risk and should be identified long before they need treatment in hospital. The arterial gases should be measured in all patients with an FEV_1 less than 1.5 l or a PEFR less than 150 l/min (Figure 3.3).

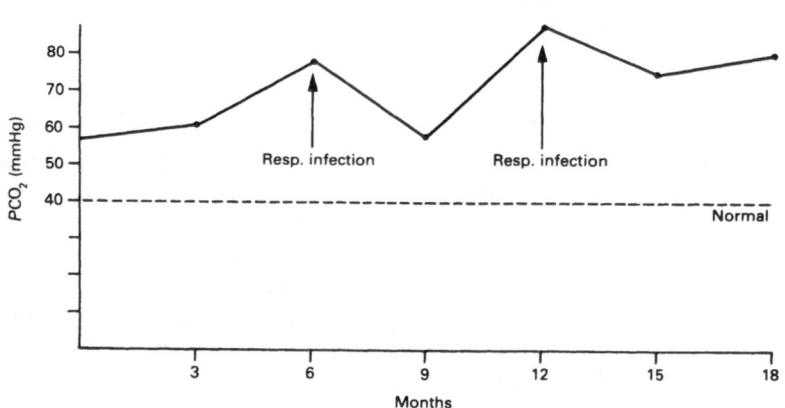

Serial measurements of arterial PCO_2 in chronic respiratory failure.

Figure 3.3

Symptoms and signs The early stages of chronic respiratory failure are easily missed because these patients are often less dyspnoeic on exertion than other chronic bronchitics with a similar degree of airflow obstruction. In more advanced respiratory failure there is cyanosis, due to a combination of hypoxia and polycythaemia. The first symptoms of hypercapnia appear when the arterial PCO_2 is above 8 kPa (60 mmHg). Common complaints are malaise, drowsiness, confusion by day and insomnia at night.

The clinical signs of severe hypercapnia are sudden jerky movements of the hands and peripheral vasodilatation indicated by a warm moist skin and bounding radial pulse. Noisy breathing and wheezing may be silenced by the grossly reduced ventilation, so that the severe airway obstruction may be overlooked. Increasing drowsiness deepens imperceptibly into coma and many of these patients die peacefully of asphyxia during the night. This is a common sequence of events in inadequately treated mild respiratory infections complicating chronic bronchitis.

Treatment
Prevention

As a result of recent statutory control of air pollution the incidence of acute respiratory illnesses during the winter months has declined in the industrial areas of the United Kingdom. The mortality from chronic bronchitis is also falling. Cigarette smoking is now the major cause of this disease which should therefore be preventable (p. 114).

Conventional breathing tests do not reveal the earliest obstructive lesions of chronic bronchitis in the peripheral airways. Other, more sensitive tests are not yet ready for general use. Patients with a chronic productive cough or a low PEFR should certainly stop smoking, though the damage is often irreversible.

Expectorants

Hypersecretion of mucus in chronic bronchitis cannot be controlled by any drug. Even atropine in doses large enough to dry the mouth is ineffective.

Expectorants are still listed in the British National Formulary. These drugs are supposed to loosen the sputum by increasing the secretion of mucus and reducing its viscosity at the same time. There is no evidence that they have more than a placebo effect. A popular remedy is a cup of tea and a cigarette on rising. A mixture of salt and sodium bicarbonate in hot water is less pleasant but works equally well.

Among the more recently introduced mucolytic drugs bromhexine (Bisolvon) has been shown to reduce the viscosity of sputum both *in vitro* and in the bronchi. This drug is least effective when most needed, during acute exacerbations with purulent sputum.

Antibiotics

Purulent sputum

Respiratory infections complicating chronic bronchitis are usually due to *Streptococcus pneumoniae*, which responds to a wide range of antibiotics, or to *H. influenzae*, with a much more narrow sensitivity spectrum. In mild infections with purulent sputum ampicillin, amoxycillin, co-trimoxazole and oxytetracycline are equally effective. A common practice is to prescribe a 5 day supply of one of these antibiotics, to be kept in reserve for self-treatment as soon as the sputum becomes purulent.

Prophylaxis

The prophylactic use of antibiotics, taken continuously during the winter, is more controversial. The results of many controlled studies agree that it does not reduce the number of infective exacerbations, though it shortens them. No antibiotic, taken prophylactically, has emerged as clearly superior to the others. These results suggest that continuous prophylaxis with antibiotics is unrewarding.

URT infections

There is no conclusive evidence that antibiotics prescribed for coryza or sore throat prevent exacerbations of chronic bronchitis. Prevention of viral infections would no doubt be beneficial, but immunization against influenza is the only practical measure available at present. Influenza vaccine (BP) 1 ml by deep subcutaneous injection is recommended for all breathless chronic bronchitics. Immunity is short lived, so that the injection must be repeated every autumn.

Flu vaccine

Bronchodilators

Performance in the forced expiratory tests usually improves after administration of bronchodilator drugs. The rise of FEV_1 and PEFR is variable and seldom as spectacular as in asthma. Bronchodilatation is accompanied by relief of dyspnoea and improved exercise tolerance, often out of proportion with the improvement shown by the breathing tests.

Beta-adrenergic aerosols

The most effective bronchodilator drugs are beta-adrenergic agonists, administered by inhalation of a single dose of aerosol delivered from a pressure packed cartridge.

Isoprenaline (Medihaler Iso), and adrenaline (Medihaler Epi) are now rarely used, having been superseded by salbutamol (Ventolin), orciprenaline (Alupent), terbutaline (Bricanyl) and rimiterol (Pulmadil). These act longer and are less likely to cause tremor and tachycardia. Comparative studies have shown only minor differences in the beneficial and unwanted effects of these drugs. Their cost is similar, so that the choice may be left to the patient's preference.

Technique The usual reason for a poor response is faulty technique of inhalation. Demonstration and training in the use of the aerosol is essential. The nozzle must be held just in front of the open mouth, and the delivery of the aerosol synchronized with the beginning of a deep inspiration. For patients who are unable to learn this simple procedure there is the choice of a cartridge containing isoprenaline, automatically triggered by inspiration (Iso-Autohaler), or salbutamol in powder form (Ventolin Rotacaps), delivered by a scattering device (Rotahaler). Bronchodilator aerosols can also be administered by nebulizer or driven into the lung by positive pressure ventilator. These methods are suitable for patients who are too weak or too dyspnoeic to take a deep breath.

Anti-cholinergic aerosols The bronchodilator effect of atropine and related anticholinergic drugs has been recognized for a long time. At first they were incorporated into medicated cigarettes, and later into aerosols, in combination with isoprenaline (PIB) or with adrenaline (Rybarvin). A test based on comparison of the bronchodilator effect of atropine with that of isoprenaline was used in the past to predict response to corticosteroids. It showed wide variation in the response to atropine between patients. Elderly chronic bronchitics generally responded better than young asthmatics.

Ipratropium Interest in atropine revived in recent years as a result of experimental work demonstrating the importance of a vagal bronchoconstrictor reflex in asthma. An aerosol containing ipratropium bromide (Atrovent) is now in general use. Comparative studies have shown that salbutamol and ipratropium together are better than either alone. Salbutamol should be prescribed first and ipratropium added later if necessary. The effect of each drug should be checked by PEFR measurements.

Oral broncho-dilators The belief that some chronic bronchitics become dependent on aerosols and inhale them in potentially lethal amounts is unjustified. Oral bronchodilator should be prescribed only for patients who cannot be taught to inhale aerosols. All these drugs have unwanted effects, particularly tremor and tachycardia.

63

Ephedrine

Oral ephedrine, and preparations containing a mixture of ephedrine, theophylline and a barbiturate (Franol, Tedral etc.) are still widely used. Apart from tremor and tachycardia ephedrine may also cause retention of urine in elderly men with prostatic obstruction. It also tends to become less effective with continued use. If an oral drug is prescribed, one of the beta-adrenergic agonists in tablet form: salbutamol (Ventolin) 4 mg, orciprenaline (Alupent) 20 mg, or terbutaline (Bricanyl) 5 mg, up to three times daily is preferable.

Salbutamol etc.

Theophylline

Theophylline might be expected, on theoretical grounds, to enhance the effect of beta-adrenergic agonists, but in practice it is often disappointing. Nausea and vomiting are common, although proprietary tablets: Phyllocontin (a slow release preparation of aminophylline) 225 mg, twice daily, or choline theophyllinate (Choledyl) 100 mg, four times daily, are better tolerated. In severe dyspnoea these drugs may be taken in addition to bronchodilator aerosols, but should be discontinued if a short trial, checked by PEFR measurements, shows them to be ineffective.

Sodium cromoglycate (Intal)

Intal is ineffective in chronic bronchitis. One of the preparations (Intal Compound) also contains isoprenaline sulphate (0.1 mg in 20 mg cromoglycate), originally intended to counteract the temporary bronchoconstriction provoked by the inhalation of a drug in powder form. This adds to the difficulty of judging whether Intal is effective because many patients report improvement that is entirely due to the bronchodilator effect of isoprenaline. Such patients should not be encouraged to persevere with isoprenaline in this expensive formulation, when many cheaper adrenergic bronchodilator drugs are available.

Corticosteroids

Many elderly chronic bronchitics take corticosteroids during exacerbations or continuously, without any beneficial effect to outweigh the potential dangers of these drugs. A few patients experience striking relief of breathlessness, with corresponding improvement of the forced expiratory tests. In some of these a previous history of episodic dyspnoea, nasal symptoms, hypersensitivity to allergens or eosinophilia help to forecast a favourable response. There remains a small minority, with clinical features indistinguishable from chronic bronchitis, whose health is dramatically and permanently improved by corticosteroids. The difficulty lies in recognizing these exceptions to the general rule that corticosteroids are ineffective in chronic bronchitis.

Trial treatment

No patient who continues to deteriorate in spite of treatment with bronchodilators and antibiotics should be denied a trial of corticosteroids. The conditions of the trial are that the corticosteroid is given in adequate dosage, for a short period only, and stopped for good as soon as the treatment has been shown to be ineffective.

The casual use of a steroid aerosol or prednisone in a daily dose of 5-10 mg by mouth is unsuitable for this purpose. Indeed no dosage schedule is perfect, but prednisone 40 mg daily by mouth for 14 days will identify most patients who benefit from long term treatment. Data concerning breathlessness, exercise tolerance, quantity of sputum and PEFR must be recorded at the start and the end of the trial. A daily record of the PEFR at 9 am and 4 pm should be kept if possible.

Often there is no subjective or objective improvement. Others report a sense of well being while taking large doses of prednisone, but on closer enquiry their dyspnoea is unchanged. The trial should then be concluded at once, without gradual reduction of the dosage.

Some patients claim to be less short of breath and support this by examples of improved exercise tolerance, but their PEFR remains unchanged. It is then justifiable to continue the trial with a lower dose of prednisone (10 mg daily) for another 4 weeks before coming to a final conclusion.

Long term corticosteroids

When a satisfactory response to the trial is beyond doubt, treatment should be continued with a corticosteroid aerosol (Becotide or Bextasol). If this is ineffective a much reduced dose of prednisone (10 mg daily) should be substituted. The dose may be increased to 30 mg daily for a few days during acute exacerbations. The remaining patients should not be given corticosteroids again and the failure of the trial should be recorded in their medical notes.

Oxygen

Although the arterial oxygen tension in chronic bronchitis is often below normal, hypoxia does not endanger life, except during severe acute infective exacerbations or in chronic respiratory failure. Dyspnoea is due mainly to the effort of breathing against an increased resistance and is seldom relieved by breathing oxygen.

O₂ in the
home

In some patients the effort of going upstairs or straining at stool is accompanied by a sharp fall of arterial oxygen tension. The increased hypoxic respiratory drive may then contribute to their distress. In these circumstances breathing oxygen for a few minutes may give some relief. For most others oxygen in the home is an expensive placebo. An oxygen cylinder and face mask may be provided only if measurements confirm the fall of arterial PO_2 during exertion.

Physiotherapy

Breathing
exercises

Some chronic bronchitics report improvement of their exercise tolerance after breathing exercises. Whether they act as a form of psychotherapy or produce a genuine improvement in respiratory efficiency is open to doubt.

The aim of these exercises is seldom stated in physiological terms. Theoretically there is an optimal rate and depth of respiration, requiring least work for a given alveolar ventilation. Advice on the correct posture of the chest and adjustment of the relative contribution of costal and diaphragmatic breathing may minimize fatigue of the respiratory muscles and improve the distribution of ventilation. The breathing pattern best suited to individual patients could in principle be discovered by elaborate respiratory measurements, but these are not suitable for clinical practice.

Relaxation

In these circumstances the effectiveness of the usual breathing exercises is at best unpredictable. They are helpful in apprehensive patients who tend to breathe rapidly when in fear of suffocation. This consumes more oxygen and may actually reduce alveolar ventilation. Instruction in relaxed breathing breaks this vicious circle.

Assisted
coughing

The most spectacular successes of physiotherapy are achieved in chest injuries and after thoracic or abdominal operations. These patients are reluctant to cough because they are weak, drowsy, breathless, or in pain. This can be overcome by vigorous persuasion. The same technique is also useful in clearing the airways of sputum during acute respiratory infections in chronic bronchitis.

Postural
drainage

The main indication for postural drainage is basal bronchiectasis, but it is also helpful in chronic bronchitis. Expiratory closure of the basal bronchi is delayed when the effect of gravity is removed in the head down posture, so that coughing becomes more effective.

PPV

Bronchodilator aerosols can be driven into the lung by

positive pressure ventilators. This method is suitable for patients who are too weak or dyspnoeic to take a deep breath. In less severely ill patients it has no special advantages.

Management of chronic respiratory failure

A common cause of death in chronic bronchitis is asphyxia from obstruction of the airways by sputum during an acute respiratory infection. In chronic respiratory failure there is an additional risk of coma from carbon dioxide retention. Unconscious patients cannot cough or co-operate in simple physiotherapy to clear their airways. This leads to a vicious circle of rising PCO_2 and deepening coma, ending in cardiac arrest from hypoxia.

The mortality amongst these patients is unnecessarily high. The first step towards more effective treatment is to recognize chronic respiratory failure by measurement of the PCO_2 in arterial blood or in gas rebreathed from an anaesthetic bag.

All respiratory infections complicating chronic respiratory failure must be treated in hospital. Arrangements should be made in advance of a crisis for automatic admission to a department where the patient is already known. Oxygen should be withheld while waiting for admission because it is likely to aggravate the hypercapnia and cause increased drowsiness or coma. All sedatives are contraindicated.

In hospital closely supervised intensive care is essential. The objective is to keep the patient awake by encouraging cough and deep breathing. Oxygen is given in low concentration not exceeding 27%. Continuous observation of the level of consciousness and frequent measurements of the arterial oxygen and carbon dioxide tension are essential. Intubation, tracheostomy and assisted ventilation should be reserved for patients whose recent history suggests that they are capable of returning to a tolerable life.

Table 3.1 Chronic bronchitis – a summary

Clinical features	
Symptoms	Cough, sputum, recurrent chest infections, breathlessness
Signs	Basal late expiratory crackles, scanty monophonic wheezes, polyphonic expiratory wheeze

Table 3.1   (Continued)

X-ray	Usually normal
Breathing tests	Low FEV_1 and PEFR. Improvement after bronchodilator aerosol
Differential diagnosis	Pulmonary tuberculosis (NB Chronic cough in elderly men should not be attributed to chronic bronchitis without a chest X-ray), bronchiectasis asthma
Complications	Pneumonia, emphysema, chronic respiratory failure, cor pulmonale
Treatment	Stop smoking. Antibiotics at the start of infective exacerbations, bronchodilator aerosols, oral aminophyllin preparations (NB Corticosteroids should not be used unless an adequate trial has proved their effectiveness.) Chest infections in chronic respiratory failure should be treated in hospital.

Asthma

Pathogenesis – Classification – Clinical features – Investigations – Differential diagnosis – Prognosis – Treatment

Definition   Asthma is easily recognized in a young patient who had eczema in infancy and now complains of paroxysmal dyspnoea with wheezing, provoked by inhaled allergens or exercise. Differences of opinion arise when persistent dyspnoea and wheezing in middle age is associated with eosinophilia and is relieved by corticosteroids. Although there is no generally agreed definition, it is widely accepted that the characteristic feature of asthma is narrowing of the intrathoracic airways (recognized by dyspnoea, wheezing or respiratory measurements), varying in severity over short periods of time. The aetiology, be it allergy or some other factor, is thus left open. It is permissible to adopt other definitions which lay more stress on hypersensitivity to allergens or response to corticosteroids, provided that the criteria are clearly stated.

Pathogenesis
Bronchial lability

Lability of bronchial calibre in patients prone to asthma can be demonstrated by an abnormally brisk response to a variety of stimuli. Histamine aerosol provokes a much greater increase of airflow resistance than in normal subjects. Inert dusts, exercise, and hyperventilation, which have a barely perceptible effect on the airways of normal subjects, often produce a sharp fall of the peak expiratory flow rate.

69

This abnormal response is due to the release of histamine and other mediators from the pulmonary mast cells. These mediators act on the airways directly and also through a vagal reflex. The distribution of calibre changes is asymmetrical, some large bronchi being narrowed to the point of closure, while others remain wide open. The behaviour of the peripheral airways in mild asthma is not well documented, but in patients who die during a severe attack they are often found to be obstructed by viscid mucus. It is probable that oedema of the mucosa, as well as contraction of bronchial smooth muscle, contributes to the airflow obstruction. The terms asthma and bronchospasm are therefore not interchangeable.

Allergy

Hypersensitivity to inhaled allergens plays an important part in the pathogenesis of asthma. A family history of allergy and associated allergic diseases, hay fever and eczema are reported by many patients. Immediate skin reactions to prick tests with allergens are much more common in asthma than in normal subjects.

Common allergens Allergens which most frequently provoke these cutaneous reactions are the house dust mite, grass pollen and extracts of the skin and fur of domestic animals, in that order. A positive skin test does not mean that the allergen is also responsible for the attacks, unless this is corroborated by the history.

Occupational asthma A relatively uncommon but important cause of asthma is exposure to allergens at work. There is a growing list of such occupational hazards, including the manufacture of drugs, detergents, plastics and resins, in addition to those previously recognized, like cotton dust, flour and contaminated grain.

Food and drink The role of food allergens in asthma is difficult to assess. In adults they play only a minor part, but in children hypersensitivity to milk, egg, fish or nuts may be more important. Attention was drawn recently to colouring agents and other additives to food and soft drinks as a potential cause of asthma. Sensitivity to alcoholic beverages is another well recognized factor. Proof is difficult and requires either provocation tests or exclusion of the suspected article from the diet.

Other factors

Drugs The aetiology of asthma in patients without evidence of hypersensitivity is obscure. Amongst drugs causing or aggravating asthma, aspirin is the most important because of its widespread use. The connection may not be recognized if the attack follows administration of a proprietary medicine containing aspirin.

A full review of the drugs taken by the patient is advisable, with particular attention to beta-adrenergic antagonists (propranolol, oxprenolol, etc.). Some drugs of this group are less likely to provoke bronchoconstriction than others, but all of them may aggravate asthma and should if possible be discontinued at least for a period of trial.

Cryptogenic asthma

In many cases no clue to the cause of the attacks can be discovered. Asthma is occasionally a presenting symptom of polyarteritis. Reports of tissue antibodies and association with other autoallergic diseases suggest that in some patients an abnormal immune response may be involved. Unhappiness, fear or anger can certainly provoke or aggravate an attack, but in the absence of other explanation the importance of emotional factors in the aetiology of asthma is easily overestimated.

Table 4.1 Asthma – pathogenesis

Bronchial lability	Exercise, hyperventilation, inert dusts
Allergy	House dust mite, grass pollen, domestic animals, occupational allergens, food and drink
Drugs	Aspirin, beta-adrenergic inhibitors (propranolol etc)
Emotional factors	
Polyarteritis	
Other autoallergies?	
Cryptogenic	

Classification

Extrinsic and intrinsic

It is customary to classify asthma as extrinsic when a history of asthma provoked by an allergen is confirmed by the prick test, and as intrinsic when there is no such evidence of hypersensitivity. Extrinsic asthma is common amongst the young, while intrinsic asthma often begins late in life. When these two groups are matched for age, most of the differences in the clinical features disappear. This method of classification is of little practical value.

Patterns of airflow obstruction

Another classification is based on the timing and duration of the attacks. 'Brittle' asthmatics are prone to chaotic variations of the peak expiratory flow rate (PEFR). They are difficult to stabilize, although individual attacks are easily relieved. The 'morning dipper' shows a regular circadian cycle of airflow obstruction, with its nadir in the early hours of the morning. This group responds poorly to corticosteroids. A third group includes patients with asthma irreversible by bronchodilators, whose PEFR is always below normal, yet varies markedly throughout the day. Many patients whose attacks begin late in life belong to this group, and they often improve on corticosteroids.

Clinical features

Presenting symptoms

The diagnosis of asthma is obvious when its presenting symptoms are short attacks of dyspnoea and wheezing in an otherwise healthy person. In its mildest form the disease may not be recognized, for example when slight wheeziness is confined to the height of the pollen season or follows prolonged strenuous exertion. It is probable that recurrent wheezy bronchitis complicating viral infections in young children is also a variant of asthma.

Duration of attacks

The length of attacks varies from short episodes of wheezing, immediately relieved by a bronchodilator aerosol, to airflow obstruction resistant to all treatment, persisting for several days.

Noisy breathing

Noisy breathing is the most constant sign of narrowing of the airways. As a general rule the loudness of the inspiratory sound at the mouth is a good quantitative sign of the severity of airflow obstruction. In asthma the noise is sometimes generated by only a few narrow bronchi, while the calibre of the other airways is normal. In such cases the inspiratory sound is louder than predicted from the FEV_1 or PEFR.

Wheezing

The number and loudness of wheezes is an unreliable guide to the severity of airflow obstruction. These sounds are generated by a few airways narrowed to the point of closure. In asthma almost complete obstruction of some bronchi is consistent with less severe narrowing or fully patent bronchi elsewhere.

72

Both large and small bronchi are capable of generating high pitched musical sounds. High pitched wheezing should therefore not be interpreted as a sign of peripheral bronchial spasm.

Danger signals   In severe asthma cyanosis, tachycardia and fading of the radial pulse during inspiration are danger signals. Wheezing is often absent in these patients and the silent chest may be misinterpreted as a reassuring sign. The absence of wheezing, profound hypoxia and poor response to bronchodilator drugs in these dangerously ill patients may be due to obstruction of the peripheral airways by viscid sputum.

Investigations

Respiratory measurements

PEFR   Clinical signs are at best a rough guide to variations in the severity of asthma. For more precise assessment instrumental measurements are essential. The most helpful test in general practice is measurement of the peak expiratory flow rate (PEFR) at the beginning of an expiration delivered with maximal force from a fully inflated chest. It often confirms the diagnosis when the history and clinical signs are ambiguous.

Exercise provocation test   If the PEFR is normal, it should be repeated after strenuous exercise. A fall by more than 20% of the previous reading, persisting for at least 30 minutes, supports the diagnosis of asthma.

Arterial gases   Arterial gas measurements are unnecessary, except during severe attacks of asthma treated in hospital. Hypoxia requiring oxygen treatment is common during these episodes, but in contrast to exacerbations of chronic bronchitis, hyperkapnia is rare. A raised PCO_2 is a sign of severe widespread airway obstruction or of extreme fatigue of the respiratory muscles calling for assisted ventilation.

Hypersensitivity tests

Skin tests   Prick tests with grass pollen and house dust extracts are used as a screening test to identify atopic patients who are readily sensitized by casual exposure to allergens. Other prick tests are helpful in confirming a history of hypersensitivity to specific allergens.

Immediate reactions   The test is performed by placing a drop of allergen extract on the flexor aspect of the forearm and gently breaking the skin surface with a tangentially held fine needle. The result is read at 15 minutes, when a weal surrounded by erythema appears in hypersensitive subjects. This immediate reaction depends on the presence of antibodies (IgE) attached to mast cells in the skin. The corresponding event in the lung, if the bronchi are also sensitized, is an attack of asthma within a minute or two after inhalation of the allergen.

Late reactions
The weal soon disappears, but in some patients a diffuse swelling develops at its site some 6–8 hours later. This late reaction is triggered by the interaction of the antigen with a precipitating antibody in the plasma. A similar late reaction in the bronchi plays an important part in allergic broncho-pulmonary aspergillosis and is also responsible for some prolonged attacks of asthma starting several hours after inhalation of an allergen. Because of the long silent period between exposure and the onset of bronchial narrowing the connection between the two events may be overlooked.

Nasal and bronchial tests
Hypersensitivity to allergens can also be demonstrated by nasal or bronchial provocation tests. They are not suitable for use in general practice because of the risk of severe bronchial reactions long after the patient has left the consulting room. When performed in hospital under close observation, bronchial provocation tests are useful in the investigation of occupational asthma.

Differential diagnosis

Chronic bronchitis
Elderly patients with a chronic productive cough, dyspnoea and wheezing are sometimes referred to clinics for an opinion as to whether their symptoms are due to chronic bronchitis or 'late onset asthma'. Some physicians believe that a high eosinophil count, nasal polypi, aspirin sensitivity and other anomalous features in a patient with a perennial cough and persistent dyspnoea are sufficient evidence of asthma. Others disagree. This is not a genuine diagnostic problem but an argument about definitions. The practical point at issue is whether such patients should be treated with corticosteroids. This question is best answered by a properly conducted therapeutic trial (p. 65).

Catarrhal children
A similar semantic problem in the guise of differential diagnosis is whether recurrent pyrexial respiratory illnesses in children with nasal catarrh, cough and wheezing are infections or asthma. The answer depends on individual opinions about the significance of positive skin tests and other indications of allergy. As far as the parents are concerned the most important point is the prognosis, which is generally favourable. The term asthma, with its alarming implications, is best avoided.

Pulmonary oedema

Pulmonary oedema is not likely to be mistaken for bronchial asthma in a patient already under observation for hypertension, myocardial infarction or valve disease. A sudden attack of severe breathlessness may however be the first indication of left ventricular failure or pulmonary venous hypertension in previously undiagnosed heart disease. The dyspnoea is due to impaired distensibility of the lung and narrowing of the bronchi by oedema of the peribronchial connective tissue sheaths. At this stage the oedema is confined to the interstitial tissue and lymphatic channels of the lung, while the alveoli and airways remain dry.

There may be wheezing, as in bronchial asthma, but a distinctive sign of interstitial pulmonary oedema is basal late-inspiratory high pitched crackling. Other clues to the diagnosis are cardiac enlargement, ankle oedema, triple rhythm and signs of a stenosed or incompetent valve.

The diagnosis is obvious in severe pulmonary oedema with flooding of the alveoli and airways. There is extreme respiratory distress, bubbling in the large airways and frothy fluid pouring from the mouth.

Tumours of the trachea and main bronchi

The first indication of a tumour in the trachea or one of the main bronchi may be dyspnoea with noisy breathing. As the narrowing approaches closure, the hissing noise at the stenosis changes to a musical sound. This is described as stridor when very loud, or wheezing when heard only close to the mouth or through the chest wall. A characteristic feature of this sign of bronchial stenosis, which distinguishes it from monophonic wheezing in asthma, is the low pitch and persistence of the sound. It is often affected by changes of posture and may be silenced temporarily by lying down or turning over in bed.

Stridor and wheezing

Spontaneous pneumothorax

Sudden increase of dyspnoea in a patient prone to episodic breathlessness may be attributed to a severe attack of asthma if the chest is not examined and the unilateral absence of the breath sounds is overlooked. Spontaneous pneumothorax complicating asthma is often due to rupture of alveoli in the depth of the lung. Air tracking along the peribronchial and perivascular connective tissue may then spread to the mediastinum as well as the visceral pleura. Surgical emphysema in the neck may be the first indication of this sequence of events and should draw attention to the possibility of unilateral or bilateral pneumonthorax.

Allergic bronchopulmonary aspergillosis

This is an uncommon cause of prolonged episodes of dyspnoea and wheezing in patients with a long previous history of asthma. Prick test with *Aspergillus fumigatus* extract produces both an immediate weal and a diffuse swelling 6 – 8 hours after the test. The blood eosinophil count is raised and specific precipitating antibodies to the fungus can be demonstrated in the serum. The sputum may contain characteristic firm yellowish-brown bronchial casts, from which the fungus can be cultured. The chest X-ray shows thick walled proximal bronchi and lobar or segmental scars left by past episodes of allergic bronchitis.

Laryngeal spasm

Nocturnal laryngeal spasm, due to aspiration of gastric contents, can be diagnosed by the history alone. These patients are awakened by intense dyspnoea due to inspiratory obstruction, accompanied by stridor. The attack lasts less than a minute and ends as abruptly as it had begun. It may be followed by a cough and scanty mucoid sputum for a few minutes. The diagnosis is confirmed by the history and X-ray evidence of gastro-oesophageal reflux.

Compulsive sighing

Compulsive sighing may be mistaken for asthma if insufficent attention is paid to the patient's account of the attacks. There is a feeling of restricted chest expansion or insufficiently deep inspiration. The discomfort reaches its peak gradually over 1 – 2 minutes and is then relieved for a time by a single deep inspiration. These cycles of dyspnoea and temporary relief often continue for some hours, especially when the patient is tired and relaxed. The diagnosis is confirmed by the characteristic spirogram (Figure 1.3).

Table 4.2 Asthma – differential diagnosis

Diagnosis	Features
Pulmonary oedema	Hypertension, aortic disease, mitral stenosis, basal inspiratory crackles
Tumour of the trachea or a main bronchus	Persistent wheeze or stridor
Spontaneous pneumothorax	Normal percussion note, absent breath sounds
Allergic bronchopulmonary aspergillosis	Bronchial casts, eosinophilia, precipitins, X-ray appearances
Laryngeal spasm	Sudden onset and end, duration less than 1 minute, stridor
Compulsive sighing	Crescendo dyspnoea, relief by deep inspiration

Prognosis

Occupational asthma

The outlook is particularly good in asthma due to avoidable allergens. This includes most cases of occupational asthma.

Children

Asthma in children usually improves with age. The attacks become progressively less frequent and often cease altogether before puberty. Some patients remain prone to episodes of dyspnoea and wheezing throughout life, but these symptoms tend to become less severe as they grow older. Remissions lasting for several years are common.

Pregnancy

The effect of pregnancy is uncertain. Some women, especially those with periodic attacks related to menstruation, are much better. In others the number and severity of the attacks is unchanged.

Late onset

The prognosis of asthma starting later in life is less satisfactory. It often begins with a series of respiratory illnesses resembling acute bronchitis. Dyspnoea and wheezing during these episodes gradually increase and the remissions tend to get shorter. Later on the clinical picture is similar to that of advanced chronic bronchitis. These patients are however less prone to chronic respiratory failure and often respond to corticosteroids. The prognosis is particularly bad when asthma starting late in life is a presenting symptom of polyarteritis.

Treatment

Mild asthma with occasional wheezing during the pollen season or after prolonged exercise needs no treatment. A bronchodilator aerosol, kept in reserve, may be useful in the event of a sudden unexpectedly severe attack. If asthma provoked by exercise interferes with games, it can be prevented by the prophylactic inhalation of a single dose of a bronchodilator aerosol.

Bronchodilator aerosols

Adrenergic drugs

In many other asthmatic patients one of the beta-adrenergic bronchodilator aerosols is sufficient to control occasional attacks. Whenever possible these drugs should be administered by pressure packed aerosol.

There is a wide choice of bronchodilator aerosols with only minor differences in potency, speed and length of action, and unwanted effects. The most rapidly acting drug, isoprenaline (Medihaler Iso) is suitable for patients prone to sudden severe attacks and for the relief of nocturnal asthma. It is effective within 5 minutes but is more likely than other beta-adrenergic drugs to cause tachycardia, anxiety and tremor.

Isoprenaline

Salbutamol etc.

For this reason one of the other, more selective bronchodilators: salbutamol (Ventolin), orciprenaline (Alupent), terbutaline (Bricanyl) or rimiterol (Pulmadil) is preferable. None of these is clearly superior to the others. All act within 15 minutes and give relief for 2 – 3 hours. The choice is a matter of individual preference. If any of them is poorly tolerated the others should be tried in turn. Aerosols containing a mixture of a beta-adrenergic drug and atropine methonitrate (Isobrovon) act longer but are not widely used.

Dangers

Mortality among young asthmatics in England and Wales rose sharply during the early 1960s. This was generally attributed to the inhalation of grossly excessive doses of isoprenaline, in a vain attempt to relieve severe asthma. The resulting mistrust of aerosols is still reflected by undue caution in prescribing.

The selective beta-adrenergic drugs in current use are less dangerous. Patients should certainly be warned not to exceed one inhalation every 4 hours, and above all, not to take additional inhalations if the first dose fails to give relief. The margin of safety with salbutamol is in fact much larger.

Anticholinergic drugs

A reflex mediated by the vagus plays an important part in bronchoconstriction triggered by the inhalation of an allergen. Animal experiments demonstrating this reflex revived interest in the use of atropin and related anticholinergic drugs in the treatment of asthma.

Ipratropium

Comparative studies of an anticholinergic aerosol containing ipratropium bromide (Atrovent) suggest that its bronchodilator effect is less predictable than that of salbutamol. At its best ipratropium is as effective as salbutamol. When used together these two drugs produce greater bronchodilatation than either alone.

In treating asthma it is best to start with salbutamol or one of the other beta-adrenergic aerosols, and to try ipratropium only if their effect is less than expected. If these drugs taken separately do not give sufficient relief they should be tried together; one inhalation of salbutamol followed 5 minutes later by one inhalation of ipratropium.

Correct use of aerosols

Training in the correct use of pressure packed aerosols is at least as important as the choice of the preparation. The mouthpiece should be held just in front of the mouth and the trigger pressed at the start of a deep inspiration. Patients who cannot perform this simple manoeuvre should try an aerosol automatically triggered by inspiration (Duo-Autohaler). Alternatively they may inhale salbutamol in powder form, dispensed in Ventolin Rotacaps and delivered by a scattering device (Rotahaler).

Oral bronchodilator drugs

If none of these preparations is acceptable, the aerosol may be replaced by an oral bronchodilator drug. The most popular

Ephedrine

preparations contain a mixture of ephedrine, theophylline and a barbiturate (Franol, Tedral, Asmapax, Amesec). There is no evidence that these drugs are superior to ephedrine alone. Ephedrine is a potent bronchodilator, but often causes tremor and tachycardia. It becomes less effective with continued use

Salbutamol

and may lead to retention of urine in elderly men. For general use tablets of salbutamol (Ventolin) 4 mg, three times daily or orciprenaline (Alupent) 20 mg, four times daily are preferable.

Theophylline

Theophylline and related drugs by mouth might be expected to enhance the bronchodilator action of beta-adrenergic aerosols. In practice they are often disappointing, partly because the absorption of oral preparations is variable. Their use is also limited by side effects, particularly nausea. This can be avoided by prescribing choline theophyllinate (Choledyl) 200 mg, or a suppository containing aminophylline 360 mg. The best time for the administration of theophylline preparations is before going to bed, to prevent nocturnal asthma.

Aminophyllin i.v.

The main indication of aminophyllin is severe asthma which does not respond to treatment with bronchodilator aerosols. Aminophylline 250 mg dissolved in 10 ml water is injected intravenously at a rate not exceeding 2 ml per minute. Rapid injection may cause cardiac arrest. This drug is effective in pulmonary oedema as well as in bronchial asthma and is particularly useful in an emergency when the diagnosis is uncertain.

Sodium cromoglycate (Intal)

This drug is a major advance in the treatment of asthma. Its mode of action is not fully understood, but it is known to inhibit the release of bronchoconstrictor mediators from the mast cells. Unlike bronchodilator drugs it gives no immediate relief in an attack, but when inhaled at regular intervals for several days at a time it is often very effective.

As a general rule Intal works well in young asthmatics who are hypersensitive to inhaled allergens. It nearly always prevents asthma provoked by exercise. It is less effective in elderly patients with no evidence of allergy, but there are many exceptions.

Intal Compound

A minor unwanted effect is occasional transient bronchoconstriction due to mechanical irritation of the bronchial mucosa by the powder particles. To counteract this, a preparation with isoprenaline sulphate 0.1 mg added to each capsule (Intal Compound) is available. A serious disadvantage of this formulation is that it increases the difficulty of assessing the effect of cromoglycate. Many patients report improvement which is entirely due to the bronchodilator effect of isoprenaline. To use Intal Compound merely as a vehicle for isoprenaline is wasteful. It should not be prescribed until the effectiveness of cromoglycate alone has been confirmed.

Indications and dosage

This drug, which is harmless and often effective, is the obvious next choice for asthmatics who cannot lead an active life or be kept comfortable on bronchodilators alone. Such patients should inhale the contents of one capsule (Intal Spincaps) four times daily from a scattering device (Spinhaler) for a trial period of at least two weeks. If complete relief, or at least marked improvement, is reported, and confirmed by measurements, treatment should be continued with a suitable dose determined by trial and error.

During remissions the dosage may be gradually reduced at fortnightly intervals and the inhalations eventually stopped altogether if the patient remains well. Training in the correct use of the Spinhaler is essential. Occasional inhalation of the drug should be discouraged because it leads to confusion about the objective of treatment. An exception is the prophylactic use of Intal in asthma provoked by exertion. A single dose of Intal inhaled one hour before exercise is an effective alternative to the prophylactic inhalation of a bronchodilator aerosol.

Corticosteroids

Mode of action
Corticosteroids act at several points on the chain of events leading to airflow obstruction in asthma. They suppress late hypersensitivity reactions and reduce the amount of bronchoconstrictor mediators released from the mast cells. Corticosteroids may also act directly on the airways, by reducing oedema of the mucosa and inhibiting the secretion of viscid mucus. As they have no immediate bronchodilator action improvement is often delayed by several hours and the full effect of treatment may not be apparent for several days.

Complications
Corticosteroids administered by mouth or injection may cause serious complications. Indigestion, haematemesis or perforation of a gastric ulcer may occur within a few days. Decalcification of bone with root pains, collapse of vertebrae and other spontaneous fractures are not uncommon during prolonged treatment with large doses. Corticosteroids may aggravate hypertension, diabetes, and reactivate tuberculosis. Other, less serious unwanted effects are obesity, hirsuties and cushingoid facies. Suppression of endogenous adrenal secretion adds to the danger of infections, accidents and emergency operations. All patients on long term oral corticosteroids should carry a card showing full details of the treatment.

Aerosols
Corticosteroid aerosols: beclomethasone dipropionate (Becotide) and betamethasone valerate (Bextasol) are free from these adverse systemic effects, as only small quantities are absorbed. Their long term effect on the bronchial mucosa cannot yet be assessed. They should be reserved for asthmatics whose

symptoms cannot be adequately controlled with bronchodilators or Intal.

Dosage The usual dose is two puffs of the aerosol four times daily. Increasing the dose or the number of inhalations has no additional effect. Becotide is available in powder form (Becotide Rotacaps), dispensed from a Rotahaler, for patients who cannot use a pressure-packed aerosol.

The length of treatment should be tailored to the pattern of the attacks. When these are frequent, or if the dyspnoea is continuous, corticosteroid aerosols should be used for an indefinite period. A cautious reduction of the number of inhalations every 6 – 12 months will show whether a remission has occurred in the meantime. Exacerbations of asthma lasting for a few days and followed by long remissions can often be controlled by a few days' treatment. Occasionally inhalations to relieve breathlessness are ineffective and should be discouraged.

Complications The only known unwanted effect of corticosteroid aerosols is oral thrush. *Candida albicans* can often be cultured from the saliva, but stomatitis, sore throat and hoarseness are uncommon provided that the dose does not exceed two inhalations four times daily. These symptoms can be relieved by local treatment with amphotericin lozenges (BPC) or undiluted nystatin mixture (BPC) four times daily.

Oral corticosteroids Oral corticosteroids should be reserved for severe asthma that cannot be controlled with bronchodilators, Intal, or a corticosteroid aerosol. Prednisone 40 mg daily is given for a few

Dosage days at a time and stopped as soon as the attack is over. It is then usually possible to continue with a corticosteroid aerosol.

Some patients with frequently recurring severe attacks need continuous treatment with prednisone. The dose should be kept as low as possible; 5 mg daily is often sufficient, while 10 mg daily is the safe upper limit for continuous treatment. The dose may be increased to 40 mg daily for two or three days at the patient's discretion during sudden exacerbations of dyspnoea which cannot be relieved with a bronchodilator aerosol. They should then revert to the usual maintenance dose. Prolonged treatment with doses in excess of 10 mg daily is dangerous, especially in elderly patients. The risks of oral corticosteroids must always be carefully weighed against their beneficial effects.

Steroid dependence Some asthmatics become dependent on oral corticosteroids and claim that any reduction of the usual dosage makes them feel ill or is followed by a relapse of severe asthma.

It is often possible to maintain these patients on a substantially lower dose, or wean them altogether by a very slow gradual reduction of the dose under cover of a corticosteroid aerosol. Reduction of the daily dose of prednisone by steps of 2.5 mg every four weeks is safe and generally acceptable. When the daily dose reaches 5 mg it should not be reduced further until the result of a tetracosactrin stimulation test shows that endogenous adrenal secretion has recovered.

Cortico-steroids in children Oral corticosteroids interfere with growth in childhood and should therefore be used with even greater reluctance than in adults. Short courses of prednisone 20 mg daily are permissible in severe persistent attacks of asthma which cannot be relieved by other means. In the few cases where severe asthma recurs as soon as oral steroids are stopped, weekly intramuscular injections of tetracosactrin acetate (Synacthen Depot) 0.5 − 1.0 ml are less likely to delay growth and are therefore preferable to continuous treatment with oral prednisone.

Choice of cortico-steroids Synthetic glucocorticoids, other than prednisone or prednisolone, are now seldom used. If indigestion is troublesome enteric coated prednisolone (Deltacortril Enteric) should be tried. A disadvantage of long-acting intramuscular injections of methylprednisolone acetate (Depo-Medrone) is that the dose cannot be varied in the short term. Triamcinolone (Ledercort, Kenalog etc.) occasionally causes steroid myopathy with weakness of the pelvic girdle muscles. Betamethasone (Betnelan) and dexamethasone (Decadron) are more expensive than prednisone without any corresponding advantages. Hydrocortisone by intravenous injection is used in the emergency treatment of severe asthma, together with intravenous aminophylline and a bronchodilator aerosol, while waiting for admission to hospital.

Hyposensitization

In hay fever associated with asthma pollen extracts (Alavac, Allpyral), given at weekly intervals over eight weeks starting in February may prevent wheezing as well as the nasal symptoms and conjunctivitis. Hyposensitization with house dust extract is ineffective. The results of trials with the more recently introduced extracts of the house dust mite (*Dermatophagoides pteronyssinus*) are also disappointing.

Mixed extracts of allergens prepared for individual patients on the basis of skin tests are widely used, but evidence of their value is entirely anecdotal. In a disease as variable as asthma selective reports of an occasional success cannot take the place of an adequately controlled trial.

Psychotherapy

Clinical experience suggests that emotional stress may precipitate an attack of asthma, while remissions are more likely in a contented frame of mind. It is seldom possible to translate these observations into effective treatment. The problems of a child who is unhappy at school can often be resolved, but adults cannot be so readily protected from domestic strife, trouble at work and the wear and tear of life. Psychotherapy in the sense of unravelling the personal difficulties of asthmatics is time consuming and unprofitable. Counselling by a doctor has no advantages over advice from a sensible friend or one of the voluntary agencies.

Fear of suffocation may lead an apprehensive patient into a vicious circle that converts a mild attack into severe asthma. Reassurance helps these patients to adopt a more economical pattern of breathing. Breathing exercises serve the same purpose by training patients to relax and moderate their efforts during attacks.

Hypnotherapy

Practitioners skilled in hypnotherapy claim good results in the treatment of asthma. The evidence was mainly anecdotal until the Research Committee of the British Thoracic Association compared the progress of two groups over a period of twelve months. One group was treated by hypnosis at monthly intervals and autohypnosis daily. The other group were taught specially devised breathing exercises aimed at relaxation. Both groups improved. In men both forms of treatment were equally effective, while in women hypnotherapy was marginally more effective than breathing exercises.

Avoidance of allergens

Occupational hazards

Where exposure to an allergen inhaled at work is the only cause of asthma, a change of occupation is unavoidable. If a dusty occupation is only one of several factors responsible for attacks the right advice depends on their relative importance and the prospects of alternative employment. Asthmatics should not smoke and in fact they seldom do. Food, drinks and drugs as potential causes of asthma are discussed on p. 70.

Domestic animals   What to do about pets is a common and difficult problem. Often there is no direct evidence that close contact with the dog or cat provokes attacks. Nevertheless their presence in the house is undesirable, especially if skin tests with their dander or fur are positive. A compromise, short of getting rid of these animals, is to board them out for a trial, thoroughly clean the house, and see if the patient's health improves.

House dust mite   The house dust mite (*Dermatophagoides pteronyssinus*) is found all over the world, particularly in mattresses, bedding and the dust of bedrooms. It likes warmth, dampness and feeds on human skin scales. Although the mite is seldom the only allergen responsible for asthma, it heads the list of allergens capable of provoking an immediate reaction to prick test in asthmatics and probably contributes to their ill health. The mites cannot be eliminated, but their number can be reduced by regular thorough vacuum cleaning of the bedroom and frequent laundering of the bedclothes.

Emergency treatment of severe asthma

Death in asthma   Severe attacks with increasing airflow obstruction resistant to bronchodilator aerosols require intensive care in hospital. Enquiries into the events leading to fatal asthma show that many patients die before or shortly after admission to hospital because the seriousness of their illness is underestimated.

Danger signals   Although an attack ending in unconsciousness or death may develop with alarming speed, there is usually time to recognize its potential danger. A history of previous severe attacks should serve as warning, especially in patients on continuous treatment with corticosteroids. A common early danger signal is failure to respond to bronchodilator drugs. A pulse rate above 120, cyanosis, fading of the radial pulse during inspiration and a PEFR below 100 l/min are other indications that immediate emergency treatment and admission to hospital are necessary.

Emergency treatment   All patients at risk of severe attacks should have a reserve supply of prednisone tablets, with instructions to take 40 mg daily for two or three days whenever their symptoms get progressively worse and fail to respond to the usual treatment.

Liaison with a hospital department where the patient is already known and is accepted at instant notice is desirable. While waiting for the ambulance aminophylline 250 mg in 10 ml water should be given by slow intravenous injection, at a rate not exceeding 2 ml per minute. Most patients will already have inhaled more than adequate amounts of a bronchodilator aerosol, so that further inhalations are likely to be ineffective. Corticosteroids have no immediate bronchodilator action, but in order to save time it is advisable to start at once with hydrocortisone sodium succinate 200 mg by intravenous injection. In asthma there is no danger of hypercapnic coma so that oxygen can be safely administered by any close fitting mask until the patient reaches hospital.

Table 4.3 Asthma – drug treatment

Bronchodilators		
Aerosols	Adrenergic	Isoprenaline, salbutamol etc.
	Anticholinergic	Ipratropium
Oral	Salbutamol, orciprenaline, ephedrine, choledyl	
Suppositories	Aminophylline	
Intal		
Corticosteroids		
Aerosols	Becotide, Bextasol	
Oral	Prednisone, prednisolone	

Emergency treatment
Intravenous aminophylline 250 mg, in 10 ml water injected at 2 ml/min;
salbutamol aerosol;
intravenous hydrocortisone hemisuccinate 200 mg;
oxygen

5 Tuberculosis

Mortality – Natural history – Presentation – Diagnostic tests –
Investigation of contacts – Prevention – Treatment

Mortality

The death rate from tuberculosis in the British Isles fell from
40 to 1 per 100 000 during the last thirty years. Most of this improvement was due to the introduction of antituberculosis
drugs. The gradual decline in mortality since the beginning of
the century reflects the rise in the standard of living, with better housing and nutrition (Figure 5.1). Figures from Western
Europe and North America show a similar trend.

At the same time tuberculosis continues to be a major
cause of ill health and death in other parts of the world. The
contrast between prosperous and poor countries is illustrated
by the high prevalence of the disease amongst immigrants from
Asia and Africa.

Natural history

The change in the natural history of tuberculous infections
since the introduction of antituberculosis drugs is equally striking. At the end of the last war, when infectious tuberculosis
Past was still widespread, most children were infected by the time
they reached puberty. Primary tuberculosis contracted in
childhood was often discovered only in retrospect by a positive
tuberculin test or calcification on the chest X-ray.

87

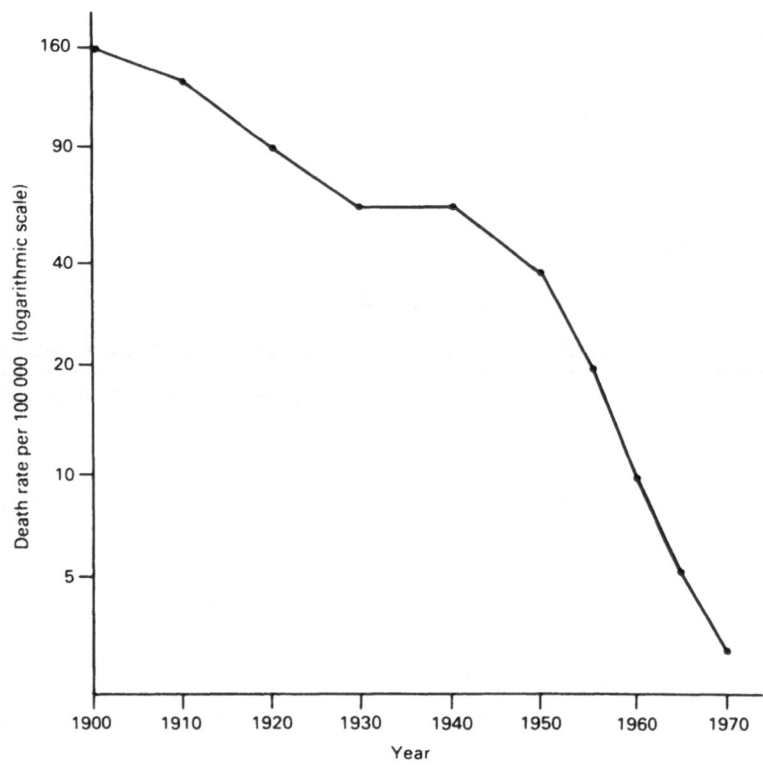

Tuberculosis mortality in England and Wales 1900–1970

Figure 5.1

Clinically manifest pulmonary tuberculosis was mainly a disease of young adults, resulting either from a recent primary infection, or from resurgence of tubercle bacilli lying dormant in the lung or the mediastinal lymph nodes since a primary infection in childhood. Mortality among adults was high and those who were apparently cured often relapsed. Infectious tuberculosis, due to reactivation of incompletely healed pulmonary lesions, was common at all ages in men, but women seldom relapsed after the menopause. Silent lymphatic or blood-borne dissemination shortly after the primary infection seeded small foci in the cervical lymph nodes, kidneys and bones. Tubercle bacilli surviving in these clinically inapparent lesions remained a potential source of extrapulmonary tuberculosis later in life.

Present   At present the main reservoir of infection in the native

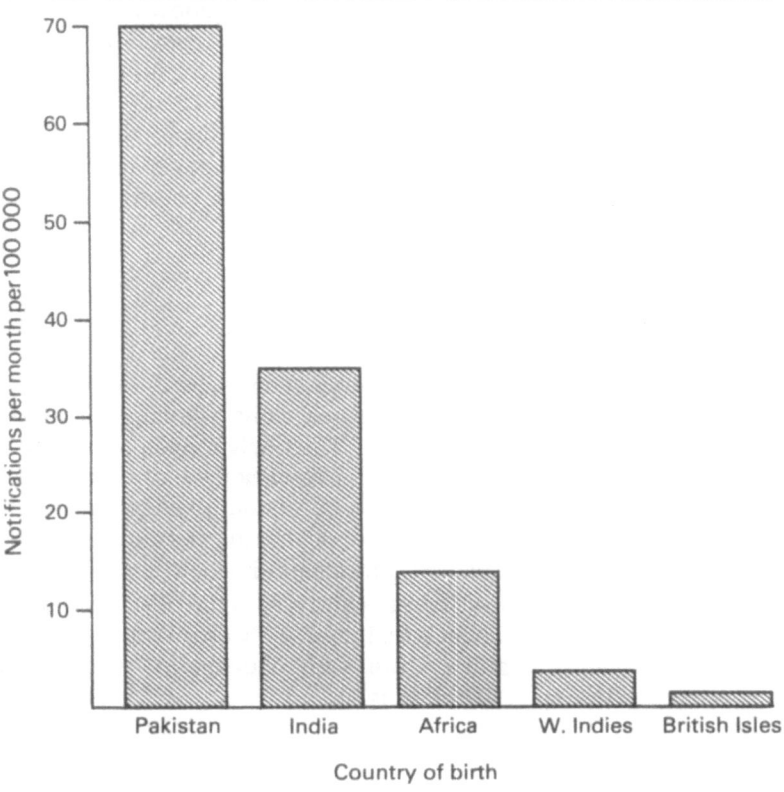

Number of tuberculosis notifications in UK per month per 100 000 population (1971)

Figure 5.2

population of western countries is undiagnosed chronic pulmonary tuberculosis in elderly men. The incidence of the disease in other age groups is falling rapidly. Nearly 90% of adolescents in Britain, tested before BCG vaccination at the age of 13 years, are now tuberculin negative. Pulmonary tuberculosis in young adults still occurs sporadically, but is diagnosed earlier and is almost always cured. In this age group tuberculosis remains a problem in alcoholics, drug addicts and other social misfits who cannot be relied on to complete their treatment. Extrapulmonary tuberculosis is even less common. It is represented mainly by elderly patients with cervical adenitis, due to the reactivation of an infection acquired several decades ago.

Immigrants   This reassuring picture does not apply to some immigrant

89

communities. A survey in 1971 showed that the tuberculosis notification rate in immigrants from Pakistan, up to 5 years after entry into the United Kingdom, was 77 times that of British-born persons. Even after 12–16 years residence their notification rate was still 46 times that of the indigenous population. The corresponding figures for immigrants from India and the new Commonwealth countries of Africa are also very high (Figure 5.2).

Presentation
Symptoms and signs

The classical presenting symptoms of pulmonary tuberculosis: loss of weight, night sweats and haemoptysis are those of acute or advanced disease. The early stages of a slowly progressive tuberculous infection are either silent or are accompanied by vague ill health and a persistent productive cough. Cough is so much more often due to smoking than to tuberculosis that it is regarded as a trivial complaint both by patient and doctor.

Most of the auscultatory signs described in the older textbooks are obsolete. Inspiratory crackling confined to the upper zones is still a useful sign, because few other diseases start in the apex of the lung.

X-ray

The early diagnosis of pulmonary tuberculosis depends on a timely chest X-ray. Unselective routine screening by annual mass radiography is no longer justifiable, but all patients attending a doctor's surgery with a persistent cough, or referred to hospital for any reason, should have a chest X-ray. Such a selective survey of people in less than perfect health remains an effective and economical method of discovering unsuspected tuberculosis.

Diabetes, chronic alcoholism and poor nutrition from any cause have long been recognized as predisposing factors. Reactivation of apparently healed tuberculosis is also one of the hazards of corticosteroid treatment. All these patients should be X-rayed at least once a year.

Tuberculosis with normal X-ray

A normal chest X-ray excludes pulmonary tuberculosis, with some exceptions. In tuberculous mediastinal adenitis a small caseous lymph node may ulcerate into a bronchus while the primary focus remains invisible. In early miliary tuberculosis the minute nodules disseminated throughout the lung

Tuberculosis

may not be apparent. The chest X-ray is sometimes normal and the tuberculin test negative in elderly patients with disseminated tuberculosis. Tubercle bacilli cannot be found in the sputum, though they are occasionally cultured from the bone marrow. Proof of the diagnosis then depends on a favourable response to antituberculosis drugs.

Another form of non-reactive tuberculosis occurs in association with pyrexia, pancytopenia and primitive white cells in blood smears. Such a leukaemoid blood picture may be due to invasion of the bone marrow by tubercle bacilli, but is more often true leukaemia complicated by disseminated tuberculosis.

Unusual presentations in immigrants

Tuberculosis in immigrants may present in forms unfamiliar to doctors whose experience of the disease is confined to Europeans. Acute disease and extrapulmonary lesions are much more common in this group.

PUO   Tuberculosis may present as pyrexia of uncertain origin. There is prolonged fever and a high ESR, without any localizing signs. The tuberculin test is strongly positive, but the chest X-ray is normal. Bacteriological and histological tests are often unrewarding. Prompt response to trial treatment with antituberculosis drugs is then the only proof of the diagnosis.

Tuberculous pneumonia   Acute pulmonary tuberculosis with clinical features resembling lobar or bronchopneumonia should always be considered in the differential diagnosis, especially in immigrants, if the infection fails to respond to antibiotics. The diagnosis is readily confirmed by a strongly positive tuberculin test and tubercle bacilli in sputum smears.

Lymphadenitis   Gross enlargement of the mediastinal or cervical lymph nodes in Europeans is likely to be neoplastic, but in immigrants it is often due to caseous lymphadenitis. Widespread enlargement of the cervical and axillary lymph nodes, suggesting reticulosis or leukaemia, may also result from lymphatic dissemination of tuberculosis. Tuberculous mesenteric lymphadenitis should be considered in the differential diagnosis of chronic abdominal pain with diarrhoea and fever.

Osteitis   Tuberculous osteitis may affect the pelvic girdle, ribs and small bones of the hands and feet, as well as the more usual sites. Pus from tuberculosis of the spine can track a long way before appearing on the surface as a subcutaneous abscess or a discharging sinus.

91

Table 5.1 Tuberculosis – unusual presentations

Acute tuberculous pneumonia
Gross enlargement of mediastinal lymph nodes
Cervical adenitis
Widespread lymphadenopathy
Chronic subcutaneous abscess
Discharging sinus
Chronic abdominal pain and diarrhoea
Pyrexia of unknown origin
Cachexia
Disseminated tuberculosis with leukaemoid blood picture
Failing health in patients under treatment with:
    cytotoxic drugs
    immunosuppressives
    corticosteroids

Delay in diagnosis

Failure to recognize tuberculosis is still all too common. An enquiry in 1968 showed that amongst 263 patients who died of active tuberculosis during a period of 3 months, the disease was diagnosed after death in 52 and was recognized too late for effective treatment in another 71. The symptoms were often attributed to chronic bronchitis or cancer. Unusual forms of tuberculosis in old people and immigrants were overlooked. A chronic cough at any age, particularly in elderly men, should not be attributed to chronic bronchitis until the chest has been X-rayed.

Diagnostic tests

X-ray appearances

Pulmonary tuberculosis can usually be recognized without supporting evidence by the distinctive pattern of shadows on the chest X-ray. Few other diseases imitate the bilateral apical distribution of mottling in blood-borne dissemination (Figure 5.3), or the combination of cavities, scarring, calcified nodules and scattered inflammatory lesions of chronic tuberculosis (Figure 5.4).

Inactive tuberculosis   It is unwise to interpret the X-ray appearances as those of healed disease without further observation. Scars and well circumscribed nodules, even when calcified, may harbour live tubercle bacilli, yet remain stable for many years. Such lesions should not be regarded as healed unless the patient has received adequate treatment in the past.

When these characteristic features are present, the

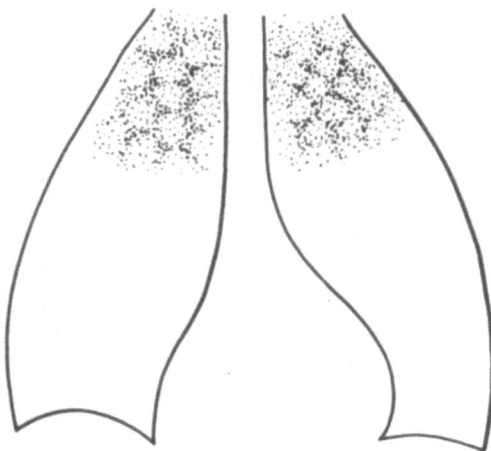

Apical mottling in blood-borne dissemination of tuberculosis

Figure 5.3

radiological diagnosis is reliable. The X-ray appearance of some other tuberculous lesions is more ambiguous. For example, miliary tuberculosis, sarcoidosis, and pneumoconiosis may look alike. Scarring of the upper lobes was often mistaken for tuberculosis before allergic bronchopulmonary aspergillosis was recognized. Dense apical non-tuberculous

Sarcoidosis
etc.

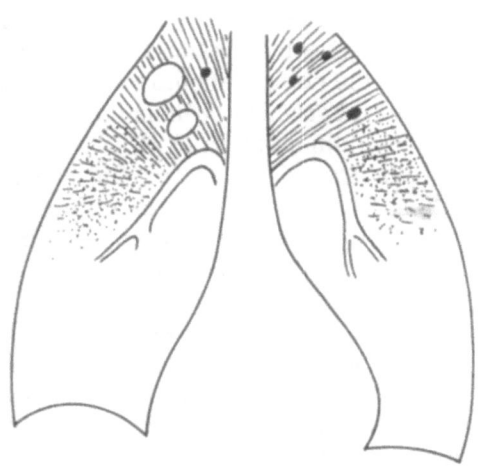

Chronic fibrocaseous tuberculosis

Figure 5.4

fibrosis also occurs in association with ankylosing spondylitis.

Tumours A common diagnostic problem is presented by an accidentally discovered small nodule in the lung. The X-ray appearance of a small malignant or benign tumour, a rheumatoid nodule and a tuberculous focus is very similar. Persistent lobar or segmental consolidation in elderly patients is usually due to obstruction by a tumour, but it may be tuberculous. The diagnosis in such cases cannot be made on radiological grounds alone.

Spread Extension of abnormal shadows in tuberculosis is usually a sign of spread of the disease. Exceptionally, in patients under treatment it may represent an allergic reaction to antituberculosis drugs. Another possible source of error is colonization of a healed tuberculous cavity by *Aspergillus fumigatus*, accompanied by an inflammatory reaction in the surrounding lung.

Sputum test

Culture Culture of *Mycobacterium tuberculosis* from the sputum proves the diagnosis. The source of the organism is nearly always visible on the chest X-ray. A positive culture should be accepted at its face value, even if no abnormal shadow is seen. Investigation of its source includes examination of the upper respiratory tract, which may reveal tuberculous laryngitis or a tuberculous ulcer in the mouth. Alternatively ulceration of a bronchus, or a sinus communicating with a caseous lymph node, may be discovered at bronchoscopy. A tuberculous lesion, invisible on a standard X-ray but demonstrated by a lateral view, is another possible explanation. Mistaken identity or contamination of the culture should not be considered until all such concealed tuberculous lesions have been excluded.

Drug-resistant strains Sputum cultures in all newly diagnosed pulmonary tuberculosis should be tested for sensitivity to antituberculosis drugs in common use. In economically advanced countries about 5% of strains isolated from the sputum before treatment are resistant to one or more of these drugs. The prevalence of primary resistance in developing countries is much higher.

Drug resistance may also develop during treatment if an unsuitable combination of drugs or an insufficient dose is prescribed, or if the drugs are not taken as directed. Sensitivity tests should be repeated if radiological progress is unsatisfactory, or tubercle bacilli persist in the sputum, and if the disease relapses after completion of treatment.

Smears Demonstration of acid fast bacilli in sputum smears is strong evidence of tuberculosis, but is not as reliable as a culture. M. *tuberculosis* and environmental mycobacteria (M. *kansasii*, M. *avium* etc.) look alike though their cultural characteristics are different.

Environmental mycobacteria
A single culture of environmental mycobacteria may be of no significance. If these organisms are repeatedly isolated from the sputum of a patient with abnormal pulmonary shadows, they are probably pathogenic. Pulmonary disease due to these uncommon infections is generally milder than tuberculosis and is not transmissible. Their identification is important because environmental mycobacteria are resistant to some of the drugs used in the treatment of tuberculosis.

Histological diagnosis

Sarcoidosis
A positive histological report can be accepted as evidence of tuberculosis even if acid fast bacilli are not seen in the sections, provided there is caseation as well as the characteristic cellular pattern. In the absence of caseation tuberculous and sarcoid lesions are very similar. The diagnosis must then be based on other clinical and radiological observations.

Cat-scratch disease
Another, uncommon source of error is infection of the axillary or cervical lymph nodes by the virus of cat-scratch disease. The histological features are similar to tuberculous adenitis. Correct diagnosis will save several months of unnecessary chemotherapy.

Tuberculin test

This test can be performed by several different methods (Mantoux, Heaf, tine). In general practice the tine test is convenient, though it gives occasional false negative results.

Tine test
The instrument is a stainless steel disc with four tines or prongs, attached to a plastic handle. The tines have been dipped in old tuberculin, dried and sterilized at the factory. They should be pressed firmly on the flexor aspect of the forearm for a few seconds. The test is read at 48–72 hours. A weal 2 mm or more in diameter at the site of one or more puncture marks is interpreted as a positive reaction. Stronger reactions range from weals merging into a circle, or a papule within or extending beyond the area bounded by the puncture marks.

Significance
The tuberculin test becomes positive 6 weeks after infection and usually remains positive for life. Its diagnostic value is limited by the fact that neither the age nor the state of healing

of the infection can be determined by the size of the reaction. As a general rule a positive reaction indicates a tuberculous infection at some time in the past, but there are some exceptions. Weak reactions may result from exposure to environmental mycobacteria. The test also becomes positive after BCG vaccination.

Adolescents responding with very large reactions to the Mantoux test are at greater than average risk of tuberculosis during the next 2 years. It is possible that this risk applies also to other age groups and to strongly positive reactions to the tine test.

With few exceptions a negative tuberculin test rules out tuberculosis. A recent infection may be missed because of a time lag of 6 weeks between infection and tuberculin conversion. Tuberculin sensitivity may be lost temporarily in infectious fevers and permanently in sarcoidosis, leukaemia and reticuloses. In acute miliary tuberculosis and in elderly patients with tuberculous cachexia the tuberculin test is often negative.

Investigation of contacts

In countries where intractable chronic tuberculosis is rare and bovine tuberculosis has been eliminated, the source of infection is usually a patient with undiagnosed pulmonary tuberculosis. Families living in overcrowded conditions are at particular risk, especially in some immigrant communities where the prevalence of the disease is high. Children are very susceptible, but infection between husband and wife is uncommon.

Procedure   When a newly diagnosed case of tuberculosis is notified, all other members of the household should be seen at a chest clinic. A tuberculin test is performed on children under the age of 13 years. If the test is negative 6 weeks after the last exposure to infection no further action need be taken. Those with a positive reaction should have a chest X-ray at once and again 6 and 12 months later.

Many adolescents and adults are tuberculin positive as a result of BCG vaccination at school. Routine tuberculin testing above the age of 13 is therefore unrewarding and a chest X-ray at the time of the first visit is sufficient. Adults sharing the same room at work should also be examined, but it is unnecessary to include other staff or casual visitors to the home.

Immigrants   In view of the high prevalence of tuberculosis in some immigrant communities the search for unrecognized disease should be more intensive. It is advisable to repeat the chest X-ray at 1 and 2 years after the first examination. The survey of contacts should include regular visitors as well as relatives and friends who have slept at the house. In districts with large immigrant populations tuberculin testing of children on entry into the primary schools might also lead to the discovery of undiagnosed infectious tuberculosis in the home.

Children with a positive tuberculin test before BCG vaccination at the age of 13 are usually referred to a chest clinic. Those with a strongly positive reaction should be kept under observation for 2 years. The others can be dismissed if the chest X-ray is normal.

Prevention

The steady fall in the death rate from tuberculosis before the introduction of chemotherapy reflects the improvement of social conditions in economically advanced countries. Better housing means less risk of infection, and improved nutrition increases resistance to progressive disease. It is also possible that natural selection has played a part in the decline of tuberculosis over a much longer period. If the present trend continues, tuberculosis will soon be eliminated from the more prosperous parts of the world.

In the meantime vigorous measures to control the disease are still necessary, especially in less favoured countries and in immigrant communities. The essentials are good housing and nutrition, early diagnosis, and efficient treatment.

BCG   The place of BCG vaccination in the control of tuberculosis is more controversial. It reduces the incidence of the disease by 80% compared with unvaccinated controls, so that it is clearly a valuable prophylactic measure in communities where tuberculosis is still common. In countries with a low and falling incidence of tuberculosis the stage will soon be reached when the number of infections prevented will be too small to justify the cost of unselective BCG vaccination.

Whatever policy is adopted, certain groups at special risk will have to be protected. These include hospital staff who come into frequent and close contact with patients. It is still customary to offer BCG vaccination to all tuberculin negative household contacts of newly diagnosed tuberculous patients. In the past, when relapse after completion of treatment was common, this was a reasonable precaution. Now that nearly all patients are permanently cured, the risk of infection ceases within a few days after the start of treatment, so that BCG vaccination of contacts is no longer important.

Chemoprophy-
laxis

There are few indications for prophylactic chemotherapy. It should be considered when a child under the age of 2 years has been in recent close contact with infectious tuberculosis. If the child was infected less than 6 weeks earlier, the tuberculin test will still be negative. The disease in this age group is so dangerous that it is justifiable to give isoniazid 5 mg/kg weight for 3 months without waiting for tuberculin conversion. An isoniazid-resistant strain of BCG is available for children who are to be immunized at the same time.

Treatment

Before the introduction of antituberculosis drugs the outcome of treatment was regarded as satisfactory when the sputum was free from tubercle bacilli and the disease, judged by X-rays, clinical signs, and the ESR, was no longer progressive. The infection was then described as inactive, quiescent, or arrested, but seldom as healed, because the risk of relapse from tubercle bacilli surviving in apparently healed lesions could not be ignored.

Objectives

The objective of treatment today is permanent cure of the infection, implying destruction of all tubercle bacilli. In principle this can always be achieved, no matter how chronic or advanced the disease, provided that an effective combination of drugs is taken in the correct dose for long enough. Failure is nearly always the result of poorly designed or executed treatment, for which the doctor or the patient may be responsible.

Indications

The indications for treatment are obvious when tubercle bacilli have been isolated or there is clinical or X-ray evidence of progressive disease. The decision is more difficult when a calcified caseous nodule or scars of an old infection are discovered on a routine X-ray in an apparently healthy person who has never received antituberculosis drugs. Such lesions may harbour live tubercle bacilli which may unexpectedly appear in the sputum or produce fresh lesions. Whether to treat these patients at once or keep them under observation until unhealed disease declares itself is a matter of opinion.

Tuberculin
positive
children

Most children and unvaccinated adolescents in economically advanced countries are tuberculin negative. It has been suggested that in this age group a positive tuberculin test by itself is sufficient evidence to justify treatment. The difficulty lies in identifying those with recent and unhealed disease.

Tuberculin positive infants and children under the age of 2 years should be treated, because the infection in this age group is necessarily recent and dangerous. In older children the primary infection may have occurred several years earlier. It may be already healed, and in any case the prognosis is favourable. The indications for treatment are therefore less compelling. The usual policy is to keep tuberculin positive children above the age of 2 years under observation for 1 year and to treat only those who develop clinical or radiological signs of tuberculosis.

Treatment schedules

There has been remarkably little disagreement about the correct choice and dosage of antituberculosis drugs or the optimum length of treatment. The recommended treatment schedules, first with streptomycin and para-aminosalicylate (PAS), later with the addition of isoniazid were generally accepted. They remained unchanged until the 1970s when they were superseded by even more effective combinations, following the introduction of rifampicin.

Standard chemotherapy
 The most effective drugs in current use are rifampicin and isoniazid. As a safeguard against the remote possibility of primary drug resistance ethambutol is added during the first two months of treatment. The following schedule is safe, effective and is well tolerated. It is generally accepted as the first choice in the treatment of all forms of tuberculosis with a 99% probability of permanent cure.

Table 5.2 Chemotherapy of tuberculosis

| Rifampicin | 600 mg* ⎫ by mouth once daily before |
| Isoniazid | 300 mg ⎭ breakfast for 9 months |

Supplemented during the first 2 months with:

| Ethambutol | 15 mg/kg weight by mouth once daily |

*The dose of rifampicin is reduced to 450 mg daily in patients weighing less than 50 kg

Although tablets containing more than one drug are generally undesirable, rifampicin and isoniazid are often given together in the form of Rimactane capsules or Rimactazid tablets. This obviates the risk that a forgetful patient might take only one of the two drugs.

Toxic effects

Isoniazid Toxic effects of isoniazid in the relatively low dose used in this schedule are very rare. Peripheral neuropathy and psychiatric disturbances have been reported, but for practical purposes the risk is negligible.

Rifampicin The hepatotoxic effect of rifampicin is enhanced by isoniazid. Liver damage, detected by a rise of serum transaminases without clinical signs, is not uncommon when these two drugs are used together. The transaminase titres usually return to normal while treatment is continued.

More severe liver damage with jaundice and hepatomegaly is rare. Rapid recovery is the rule when treatment is temporarily stopped.

Hypersensitivity reactions with thrombocytopenia or fever, headache and muscle pains, resembling influenza, are very uncommon when rifampicin is taken daily. They are more frequent when larger doses of rifampicin are taken once or twice a week. For this reason intermittent regimens containing rifampicin are unsuitable for general use.

Cutaneous hypersensitivity reactions with flushing, itching or a rash are more common, but they are benign and respond to treatment with antihistamines or temporary interruption of treatment. Patients should be reassured before starting treatment that discoloration of the urine by rifampicin is harmless.

Oral contraceptives may be inactivated by rifampicin.

Ethambutol Ethambutol is well tolerated and is for practical purposes free from toxic effects. Early reports suggested that retrobulbar neuritis might be a serious hazard, but this was not confirmed by wider clinical experience. The recommended dose of 15 mg/kg weight should however not be exceeded and patients should be warned to report dimness or blurring of vision. In the absence of these symptoms routine ophthalmoscopy and visual field tests are unnecessary.

Supervision

Tubercle bacilli become resistant to any drug unless a suitable companion drug is taken at the same time. Frequent interruption of treatment or réduction of the dose may have the same effect. Rigid adherence to the prescribed treatment schedule is therefore essential.

100

Tuberculosis

In order to ensure compliance, the early stages of treatment should be closely supervised. Patients should be seen at least once a week during the first month, so that misunderstanding, intolerance and unwanted effects can be remedied at once. Those who for one reason or another cannot be relied on to follow instructions should be visited frequently by the district nurse. Patients whose past treatment record is unsatisfactory should have their drugs dispensed daily at home or at a clinic.

An alternative treatment schedule, suitable for uncooperative patients requiring close supervision, is streptomycin 0.75 – 1.0 g by intramuscular injection and isoniazid 800 mg (or 14 mg/kg weight) by mouth, twice weekly. Peripheral neuropathy on this high dose of isoniazid can be prevented with pyridoxin 10 mg by mouth daily.

Hospital

Dangerously ill patients and those living in poor conditions should be admitted to hospital. For others, treatment at home is equally satisfactory. The effect of bed rest, fresh air, good food and the traditional amenities of sanatoria is negligible in comparison with that of antituberculosis drugs.

Protection of the family was one of the reasons in the past for admitting patients into hospital. Isolation has become less important since the introduction of antituberculosis drugs. The risk of infection to close contacts falls sharply within a few days of starting treatment, even when tubercle bacilli are still present in the sputum. A short stay in hospital might still be advisable for patients in close contact with young children. The traditional precautions in the home, including segregation of married couples, are no longer necessary.

Drug resistant infections

These reassuring observations on the safety of domiciliary treatment do not apply to infections with drug resistant strains of *M. tuberculosis*. With few exceptions these patients have already been treated unsuccessfully on one or more previous occasions. The usual reason for failure is inadequate treatment: drugs taken singly, or with an unsuitable companion drug, or in an insufficient dose. Although this is not always the patient's fault, lack of co-operation is by far the most important factor.

101

This group includes a large proportion of alcoholics, drug addicts, vagrants and other psychiatric problems. Successful treatment in these circumstances depends on careful selection of the right drugs, which must be administered under direct supervision. For this reason, and also in order to safeguard contacts from the danger of infection with a drug resistant strain, admission to the isolation ward of a hospital is essential.

Reserve drugs   Drugs held in reserve for the treatment of infections by resistant strains are pyrazinamide, cycloserine, ethionamide, thiacetazone, PAS, viomycin and capreomycin. Some of these have only weak antituberculosis action, others are poorly tolerated and most of them are likely to cause toxic reactions. With the exception of pyranizamide they are not used in primary treatment.

The choice of the best combination, in the light of bacteriological reports on drug sensitivity, is a task for physicians experienced in the treatment of tuberculosis. Successful treatment depends on close supervision, constant encouragement and skilled management of toxic reactions. The disastrous implications of failure often leave no alternative to a stay of several months in hospital.

Extrapulmonary tuberculosis

Tuberculosis of the cervical lymph nodes, bones and the genito-urinary tract should be treated on the same lines as pulmonary tuberculosis. Experience with lung infections has shown that tubercle bacilli often survive in caseous lesions long after they have disappeared from the sputum, even when the infection appears to be clinically and radiologically healed. There is no reason to believe that tubercle bacilli in extrapulmonary lesions are any more vulnerable to drugs. It is therefore just as important to continue chemotherapy for at least 9 months.

Suppuration in tuberculous lymph nodes and bones may continue in spite of effective chemotherapy, so that an abscess or a sinus sometimes appears after the start of treatment. Such complications should not be regarded as evidence of failure. Suppuration may result from a tissue reaction to tuberculoproteins and does not necessarily depend on continued multiplication of tubercle bacilli.

Surgical treatment   Tuberculous abscesses in lymph nodes, bones and the genito-urinary tract, which fail to resolve or grow larger in spite of chemotherapy, require excision of necrotic tissue.

102

Tuberculosis

There are few indications for surgical treatment in pulmonary tuberculosis. Resection of destroyed lobes, caseous masses and cavities is unnecessary now that they can be sterilized with antituberculosis drugs. An isolated lesion, harbouring drug resistant tubercle bacilli, may occasionally need resection.

Observation

It was customary in the past to keep patients with apparently healed tuberculosis under observation for many years. Relapse after chemotherapy is now so rare that regular attendance at the chest clinic may be stopped one year after completion of treatment. Continued observation is advisable when there are grounds for suspecting that the drugs were not taken regularly. Elderly men with pulmonary lesions of doubtful state of healing who never received antituberculosis drugs should also be kept under observation.

Cancer of the lung

Mortality – Aetiology – Classification – Presentation – Clinical
signs – Progress – Investigations – Differential diagnosis –
Prevention – Treatment

Mortality

The alarming increase in the prevalence of cancer of the lung
during the last few decades is well documented and is also obvious to any practising physician. In 1977 it killed 27 000 men
and 7000 women in England and Wales alone and is now the
most common malignant tumour in men. A similar trend has
been reported from many other economically advanced countries, though the mortality figures for Great Britain are still the
highest in the world. Although cancer of the lung is mainly a
disease of elderly men, there is no comfort in the statistics,
which show that its prevalence among women is rising and that
about 40% of its victims die before reaching the age of 65.

Aetiology

Smoking The evidence incriminating cigarettes as the chief cause of carcinoma of the bronchus is overwhelming. This was first
recognized 40 years ago and since then many reports from
Europe and North America confirmed the close correlation between the number of cigarettes smoked and the risk of developing cancer of the lung. A prospective study of British doctors,
which incidentally confirmed this correlation, is of particular

interest. Most of the smokers gave up cigarettes in the course of this 20 year study. The death rate from lung cancer among doctors fell steeply during this period, while in the rest of the population it continued to rise.

Other factors

Atmospheric pollution plays an additional part in the aetiology of lung cancer. There is also an occupational risk from several industrial dusts, including asbestos. The contribution of these hazards, compared with tobacco smoking, is relatively small. Amongst the different histological types only the relatively uncommon bronchial adenocarcinomata and alveolar cell tumours are unrelated to inhaled carcinogens.

Classification

Histological varieties

Nearly all malignant tumours of the lung arise from bronchial epithelial cells. About half of these are squamous cell carcinomata, a well differentiated and relatively slowly growing variety. The other common histological type, representing about one third of all lung cancers, is an anaplastic tumour, consisting either of small cells resembling lymphocytes (oat cells), or of large undifferentiated cells. These grow and disseminate more rapidly and their prognosis is poor. Other, less common varieties are adenocarcinomata and tumours arising from the alveolar epithelium.

Site

About 50% of tumours, particularly squamous cell carcinomata, lie in the principal, lobar or segmental bronchi. Both central and peripheral tumours may spread through the lymphatic channels to the mediastinal nodes and the pleura, and disseminate by the blood stream to distant sites, especially the brain, liver and bones. Histological classification is important, not only in relation to prognosis, but also in the selection of patients for surgical treatment.

Presentation

Silent tumours

Cancer of the lung is often discovered by routine radiography in an apparently healthy person. These are usually peripheral tumours, casting a small round shadow. The differential diagnosis between a tuberculous focus and a benign or malignant tumour is difficult and frequently rests on radiological evidence alone. Calcification on plain films or tomograms suggests tuberculosis or a benign tumour. Comparison with earlier films may provide information about the age and rate of growth of the nodule.

An essential investigation is examination of the sputum for

tubercle bacilli and malignant cells. Some of these accidentally discovered nodules lie within the range of the bronchoscope. In other cases a biopsy forceps or a bronchial brush can be advanced to the nodule under radiographic control. A more hazardous method of obtaining biopsy material is transpleural needle biopsy. If the patient is young and fit, and the diagnosis is still uncertain, thoracotomy is justifiable in the last resort.

Symptoms

Cough   A mild productive cough is so common in elderly smokers that it seldom arouses suspicion in the early stages of cancer. Later on, when the cough becomes paroxysmal and keeps the patient awake at night, it is no longer likely to be mistaken for a smoker's cough. By then a major bronchus is usually occluded and the lung beyond it is atelectatic.

Haemoptysis   Blood staining of the sputum is a common presenting symptom of lung cancer. Its diagnostic value is obscured by the fact that blood, mixed with purulent sputum, is often reported during infective exacerbations of chronic bronchitis. A single episode of this kind needs no immediate action. But recurrent bleeding, or blood stained sputum in the absence of a bronchial infection, requires full investigation, including bronchoscopy.

Dyspnoea and wheezing   Persistent wheezing with increasing dyspnoea gives early warning of impending obstruction of a major bronchus. Some observant patients notice that the wheeze is unilateral and that it can be silenced by changes of posture. Increasing breathlessness may also be a symptom of a silently accumulating large pleural effusion, or compression of the central bronchi by enlarged mediastinal lymph nodes. Occlusion of a major bronchus, with atelectasis of the obstructed territory of the lung, is often accompanied by sudden breathlessness and chest pain.

Pneumonia   The first indication of a bronchial carcinoma may be an acute infection of the lobe served by a narrowed bronchus. Its clinical features are similar to those of primary lobar pneumonia. If the bronchus is not completely occluded, the consolidation resolves under treatment, but soon recurs. In others the persistence of sputum, delayed resolution, or an abscess in the obstructed lobe draws attention to the tumour. The pulmonary infection may be accompanied by a pleural effusion which clears up on antibiotic treatment. Such effusions are inflammatory and should not be regarded as evidence of a disseminated inoperable tumour.

Pain   Chest pain may be the presenting symptom of a peripheral tumour infiltrating the chest wall. Apical tumours eroding the first rib and infiltrating the brachial plexus cause severe shoulder pain radiating down the arm.

Mediastinal obstruction   In others the first indication of cancer is involvement of the mediastinal lymph nodes with obstruction of the superior vena cava, dysphagia, or hoarseness due to paralysis of the left recurrent laryngeal nerve.

Distant metastases   A tumour of the lung may metastasize to distant organs before the primary tumour is large enough to cause any symptom referred to the chest. Many cerebral tumours investigated in neurosurgical departments prove to be secondary to a carcinoma of the bronchus. Spinal metastases may present with sudden back pain or paraplegia in a patient who is apparently in good health. In many others loss of weight, cachexia, jaundice and other symptoms of extensive dissemination are the first indication of cancer.

Hypertrophic osteo-arthropathy

Painful swelling of the wrists and ankles, with radiological evidence of periosteal new bone formation, is occasionally the first manifestation of a latent carcinoma of the bronchus. These symptoms subside immediately after removal of the tumour. Division of the vagus or a simple thoracotomy is often followed by prompt relief of the joint pains, even when the tumour proves to be inoperable.

Neurological syndromes

Several non-metastatic neuromuscular syndromes have been reported in association with malignant tumours, particularly with small cell carcinoma of the bronchus. Their pathogenesis is obscure. The most common syndrome is a sensory neuropathy with paraesthesiae in the hands and feet. Other neurological complications include cerebellar ataxia, progressive dementia and various myopathies. One of these resembles myasthenia gravis, but spares the facial and ocular muscles and does not respond to edrophonium (Tensilon).

Endocrine syndromes

Hormones secreted by anaplastic tumour cells may imitate almost any endocrine disorder. As a rule these endocrine syndromes are late complications which aggravate the patient's suffering or hasten his end, but they may also be the first manifestation of cancer. The associated biochemical disturbances may respond to appropriate treatment even when the tumour cannot be removed.

Cushing syndrome

Amongst the endocrine effects of carcinoma of the bronchus the most common one is adrenal hyperplasia with potassium depletion and muscle weakness, followed by a fully developed Cushing syndrome. It is due to ectopic secretion of a polypeptide similar to ACTH. The electrolyte disturbance may respond to treatment with spironolactone and potassium.

Water retention

Ectopic production of antidiuretic hormone results in water retention with low serum sodium and secretion of concentrated urine. The resulting cerebral oedema may be mistaken for intracranial metastases. Its symptoms,

Table 6.1 Cancer – presentation

Silent tumour discovered by X-ray	
Respiratory symptoms:	Cough
	Haemoptysis
	Dyspnoea
	Wheezing
	Pneumonia
Metastases:	Pleural effusion
	Chest or shoulder pain
	Mediastinal obstruction
	Cerebral tumour
	Spinal compression
	Loss of weight
	Cachexia
	Jaundice
Systemic manifestations	Hypertrophic osteoarthropathy
Neurological:	Polyneuropathy
	Motor neurone disease
	Myopathy
	Myasthenia
	Cerebellar ataxia
	Dementia
Endocrine:	Cushing syndrome
	Water retention
	Hypercalcaemia

drowsiness and confusion, can be relieved by water restriction and fludrocortisone (Florinef) 5 mg daily by mouth.

Hyper-
calcaemia
Both these syndromes are peculiar to small cell carcinoma, while hypercalcaemia is more common in squamous cell tumours. It may be due to osteolytic metastases, but can also result from ectopic secretion of parathyroid hormone. The symptoms, thirst, anorexia, constipation and mental confusion, often respond to treatment with phosphates by mouth or intravenous infusion.

Clinical signs

Consolidation
A tumour surrounded by aerated lung tissue cannot be detected by clinical examination. Obstruction of a major bronchus is revealed by the usual signs of consolidation or atelectasis. Severe bronchial narrowing, just short of occlusion, may be accompanied by a wheeze, containing a single low pitched musical note. Characteristic features of this monophonic wheeze are its persistence, fixed pitch and sensitivity to change of posture.

Clubbing
Clubbing of the fingers may be the first sign of a small peripheral tumour, long before it produces respiratory symptoms. Clubbing may also appear later as a sign of suppurative pneumonia or empyema complicating obstruction of a major bronchus.

Lymph nodes
The cervical lymph nodes should always be carefully examined. One of the earliest signs of dissemination, a single hard nodule behind the head of the clavicle, is easily missed.

Mediastinal
obstruction
Infiltration of the mediastinal lymph nodes with obstruction of the superior vena cava is accompanied by engorgement of the superficial neck veins, oedema of the face and cyanosis. Horner's syndrome indicates involvement of the inferior cervical sympathetic ganglion by an apical tumour.

Hepatomegaly
Examination of the abdomen may reveal an enlarged hard nodular liver as the only sign of a widely disseminated growth.

Progress

Few untreated patients survive longer than one year from the time of diagnosis. Anaplastic tumours, especially small cell carcinomata, run a more rapid course and disseminate earlier than well differentiated squamous cell tumours. There is progressive loss of weight with increasing weakness, but the disease is often painless to the end.

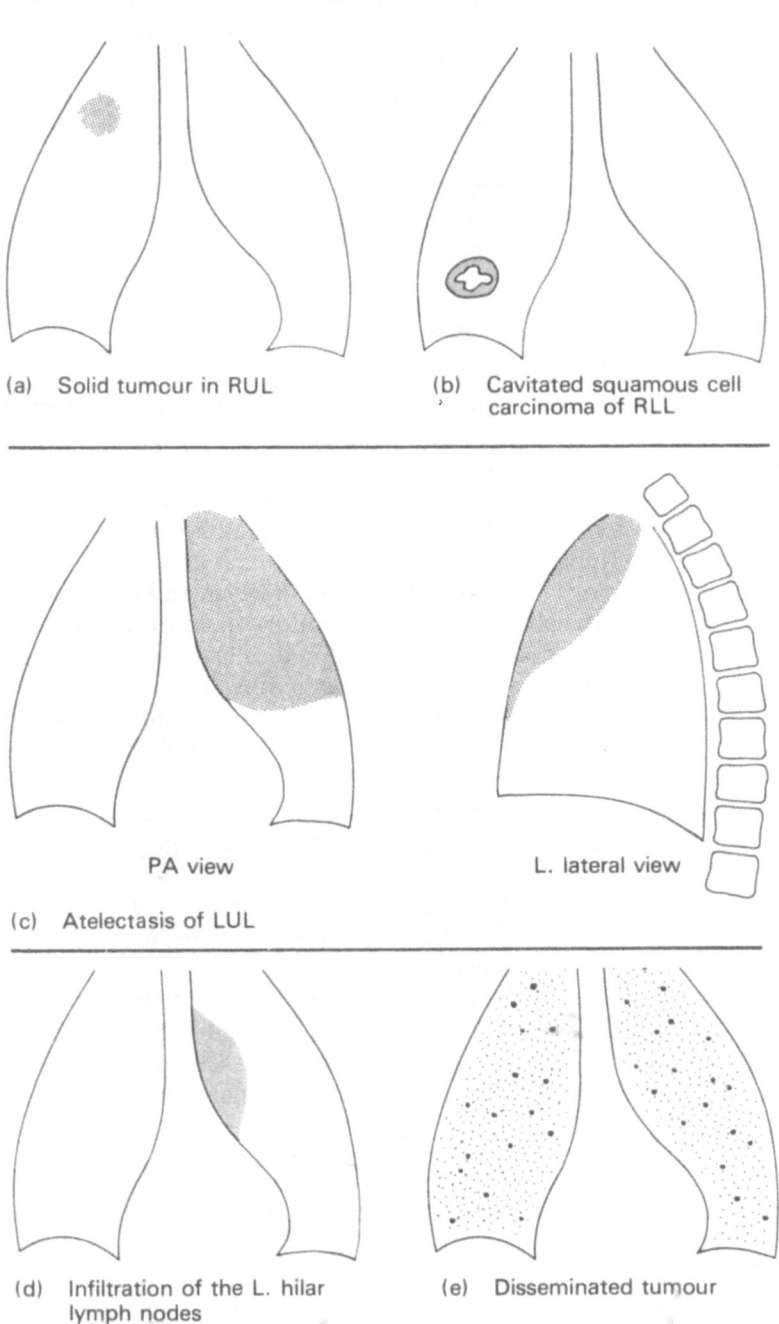

(a) Solid tumour in RUL

(b) Cavitated squamous cell
carcinoma of RLL

PA view

L. lateral view

(c) Atelectasis of LUL

(d) Infiltration of the L. hilar
lymph nodes

(e) Disseminated tumour

Figure 6.1

In others palliative treatment is required for pain due to infiltration of the chest wall or to spinal metastases. Massive involvement of the mediastinal lymph nodes is responsible for some of the most distressing symptoms: severe dyspnoea from tracheal compression, dysphagia, and obstruction of the superior vena cava. The immediate cause of death is often a respiratory infection. Occasionally death is sudden from a large haemoptysis, pulmonary embolism or mediastinal obstruction.

Investigations
X-rays

Round shadows
Large intrapulmonary tumours cast a uniformly dense shadow with clear cut or shaggy margin (Figure 6.1a). Some necrotic squamous cell carcinomata are cavitated in the centre. These resemble an abscess, but are surrounded by a wall of irregular width and there is no inflammatory reaction in the surrounding lung (Figure 6.1b).

Consolidation
An obstructed lobe is airless and uniformly opaque. If the alveoli fill with inflammatory exudate the lobe retains its normal dimensions. Usually there is some shrinkage, compensated by distension of the adjoining lobe and displacement of the mediastinum (Figure 6.1c). Overdistension of the left upper lobe may be the only clue to a shrunken left lower lobe hidden behind the heart.

Dissemination
The tumour may still be invisible when the hilar lymph nodes are already infiltrated. A large hilar shadow is then the only radiological sign of cancer (Figure 6.1d). In others an invisible tumour can be inferred from a raised immobile diaphragm, due to phrenic paralysis, erosion of a rib, or a large silent pleural effusion.

Widespread dissemination of the tumour produces nodules or reticulation throughout the lung (Figure 6.1e). Such appearances are often described as lymphangitis carcinomatosa, although the dissemination is usually blood-borne.

Bronchoscopy

The traditional rigid bronchoscope is being superseded by a flexible fibreoptic instrument, which can be introduced under local anaesthesia and offers a wider range of vision. Conventional bronchoscopy under general anaesthesia, performed by an experienced operator, is quicker and less distressing. For patients who might be suitable for surgical treatment it is the method of choice.

All accessible branches of the bronchial tree are examined and if the tumour is visible a small fragment is removed with a biopsy forceps for histological examination. Biopsy material from tumours lying beyond the range of the bronchoscope can be taken with a fine forceps or a brush, introduced under radiological guidance.

The bronchi are always inspected for signs of dissemination. Distortion of the carina and compression or rigidity of the main bronchi are signs of spread to the mediastinal lymph nodes.

Sputum cytology

Examination of the sputum for malignant cells is particularly useful when the tumour lies beyond the range of the bronchoscope, and in patients who are too old or too ill for any invasive investigation. Departments specializing in sputum cytology correctly diagnose cancer in 70% of cases if three specimens are submitted. If only one specimen is examined the success rate is 50%. False positive results are rare.

A positive cytological report by an experienced pathologist may be accepted as proof of the diagnosis. In patients who are unsuitable for surgical treatment no further investigation is necessary.

Mediastinoscopy

This uncomfortable investigation, carried out through a suprasternal incision, should be reserved for patients who appear to be suitable for surgical treatment. If the upper mediastinal lymph nodes are infiltrated the tumour is inoperable.

Transpleural needle biopsy

The risks of transpleural needle biopsy include pneumothorax, which can be foreseen and treated. Haemorrhage from a large blood vessel is a more serious complication, responsible for occasional deaths. This procedure is justifiable only when an undiagnosed nodule in the lung is thought to be a malignant tumour suitable for resection. The alternative is exploratory thoracotomy with immediate histological examination of a frozen section.

Differential diagnosis

Tuberculosis   If an accidentally discovered solitary nodule proves to be a tuberculous granuloma or a caseous focus at thoracotomy, no irreparable harm will have been done, except for an unnecessary operation. A more serious mistake is to attribute lobar or segmental consolidation in old age to an inoperable tumour without formal proof of the diagnosis. The bronchial obstruction may be due to a tuberculous lesion which is easily curable by chemotherapy.

Cancer of the lung and pulmonary tuberculosis occur together more often than expected from chance coincidence. Pyogenic infection in a lobe obstructed by a tumour may reactivate a dormant tuberculous lesion. Alternatively a tumour may start in the scar of an old tuberculous infection. A report of tubercle bacilli in the sputum should therefore not end the investigations if cancer seems likely on clinical or radiological grounds.

Metastatic tumours   The X-ray appearance of a single blood-borne metastasis from a tumour of the kidney, thyroid or stomach may be indistinguishable from a primary lung tumour. A reticuloma involving the mediastinal lymph nodes may be mistaken for infiltration by cancer of the lung. A correct histological diagnosis is important because some of these tumours respond to irradiation or chemotherapy.

Benign tumours   Tumours of relatively low malignancy (bronchial adenoma) and benign tumours (hamartoma) are rare. They represent about 1% of all pulmonary neoplasms. Bronchial adenoma may present with a frank haemoptysis, but is often silent until it obstructs the bronchus. These tumours are frequently within range of the bronchoscope. Hamartomata usually lie more peripherally. One of their distinctive radiological features is a small speck of calcification within a well circumscribed round shadow.

Prevention
Smoking

Tobacco smoking is by far the most important cause of lung cancer. There is no prospect of improvement while cigarette consumption remains at its present level.

Tobacco was introduced into Britain in the 16th century, shortly after the discovery of America, where it was widely used by the Indians. Pipe smoking, tobacco chewing and snuff were gradually overtaken by cigarettes after the First World

114

War. By 1960 over 60% of men were regular cigarette smokers and only 5% were smoking pipes or cigars. Smoking by women was socially unacceptable until the 1920s. Since then increasing numbers have taken to cigarettes, reaching 40% by 1960. In the last 20 years the percentage of male smokers has fallen by 15%, while in women the percentage remains unchanged.

Tobacco dependence

The pleasures of smoking include the familiar ritual of lighting up, the taste and smell of smoke, and above all the pharmacological effects of the various chemicals contained in tobacco, amongst which nicotine is the most important. Many smokers become dependent on tobacco and suffer from physical and mental withdrawal symptoms when deprived of their usual daily ration. As in other forms of drug dependence the habit is difficult to break. Most smokers try at some time or other but few do so permanently.

Mortality

The disastrous consequences of this mass addiction were recognized only in the last 40 years. Three of the major respiratory diseases: cancer of the lung, chronic bronchitis and emphysema are almost entirely the result of cigarette smoking. It is also an important contributory factor in coronary artery disease. About 25 000 lives are lost every year in the age group 35 – 64, as a result of smoking. This is comparable with the mortality figures of the epidemic fevers of the past and greatly exceeds the number of deaths on the roads.

Preventive measures

A problem of this magnitude cannot be solved by individual effort alone. Like other major health hazards of the past it requires concerted action by publicity, education and legislation. A series of reports by the Royal College of Physicians of London outlines the measures proposed for the control of smoking. Each of the first two reports, in 1962 and 1971, was followed by a small drop in the number of male cigarette smokers, but few of its recommendations for official action were put into practice. It is too early to judge the effect of the latest report on 'Smoking or Health', published in 1977, which is essential reading for everyone concerned about this unnecessary loss of life.

Advice by doctors

Doctors are in a favourable position to make individual contributions to the control of smoking. Patients are in a receptive frame of mind when they are worried about their health and are more likely to stop smoking if a doctor advises them to do so. Such advice should be given firmly and without reservation to patients with a chronic cough or breathlessness, and in coronary or peripheral artery disease. In diseases less closely related to smoking it is sufficient to point out the harmful ef-

115

fects of smoking on health and to leave the decision to the patient. The facts about cancer, bronchitis, cardiovascular disease, shorter expectation of life, the adverse effects of smoking on the baby in pregnancy, and on physical fitness in general should be clearly stated.

Therapy

Many patients wish to stop smoking, but have either failed in the past or lack the will to do so. They often ask the doctor for help in the form of some medication or psychological treatment. Chewing gum containing nicotine (Nicorette) is successful in about one third of cases. Other drugs like lobeline are ineffective. Some successes have been reported after aversion therapy by rapid smoking or electric shock, but the specific effect of these time consuming and unpleasant techniques is doubtful, compared with simple repeated intensive persuasion. Hypnosis, like other forms of individual psychotherapy, may also succeed in selected subjects but is unsuitable for general use. Group therapy in smoking withdrawal clinics is gaining ground, but there is little published information about their results. Their success is evidently not spectacular; only one in five of their clients stop smoking for more than a year. This is not much better than the 14% success rate at 2 years amongst those who have given up smoking by their own unaided efforts.

Change of smoking habits

If total abstinence from tobacco is rejected or has been tried and failed, a change to less harmful smoking habits is better than nothing. Some patients try to compromise by offering to reduce their cigarette consumption. This is almost invariably unsuccessful in the long run.

Since lung cancer is probably caused by a carcinogen in the tar fraction of smoke, it is reasonable to recommend a change to filter tipped cigarettes or to a low tar brand. A possible source of failure with low tar cigarettes is that they also contain less nicotine, which is probably the drug responsible for physical dependence on tobacco. It is therefore possible that some patients make up the deficiency, when changing to a low tar brand, by increasing their cigarette consumption. The harmful ingredient in coronary disease is carbon monoxide as well as nicotine, so that low tar cigarettes have no advantages for this group of patients.

Pipe smoking and cigars are less dangerous than cigarettes, though the risk of lung cancer is still higher than in non-smokers. It would seem to be reasonable to recommend a change to these less harmful forms of smoking to those who cannot live without tobacco. But these reassuring observations apply only to veteran pipe and cigar smokers who do not inhale. A cigarette smoker may continue to inhale when changing to a pipe or cigars and thereby increase the risk of bronchitis and cancer.

Treatment
Surgery

Results Lobectomy or pneumonectomy offers the best chance of cure. It is a poor best, because only one in five patients is suitable for resection and less than one third of these are alive 5 years after the operation. The overall 5 year survival rate is thus between 5 and 10%.

Contra-indications Many patients are too old, ill or breathless even to be considered for thoracotomy. Others prove to be unsuitable on investigation, for a variety of reasons. Dissemination of the growth, indicated by palpable cervical lymph nodes, hepatomegaly and metastases in bone, are obvious contraindications. Invasion of the mediastinal lymph nodes detected by X-ray, bronchoscopy or mediastinoscopy, phrenic or laryngeal paresis, and tumours lying too close to the bifurcation of the trachea, are other evidence of an inoperable tumour.

Infiltration of the chest wall, brachial plexus, or the inferior cervical sympathetic ganglion (Horner's syndrome) are also contraindications. So is a pleural effusion, unless it can be shown to be secondary to infection of the underlying lung and not to carcinomatosis of the pleura. The results of surgery in anaplastic small cell (oat cell) tumours are so poor that they are seldom referred to thoracic surgeons. Even after this strict selection procedure many tumours are found to be inoperable at thoracotomy.

Radiotherapy

There are few controlled studies of radiotherapy as the first choice for operable tumours. In one study of squamous cell carcinoma the 4 year survival rate was much lower (6%) than for resection (30%). In small cell anaplastic carcinoma the results of both forms of treatment were very poor, but the 5 year survival rate after radiotherapy (5%) was slightly better than the survival rate after resection (1%).

Radical In inoperable tumours the beneficial and adverse effects of radical radiotherapy must be carefully weighed. Most patients feel ill while under treatment, and some develop symptoms of radiation damage to the lung or oesophagus. Tem-

117

porary remission of the growth is common, but there is no evidence of longer survival.

Many doctors and most families feel that an attempt should be made to save the patient's life. Radical radiotherapy cannot do so and should therefore not be advised lightly. It is however reasonable to recommend it for small localized tumours when surgery is not possible because of breathlessness, age, or poor health. There is no evidence that irradiation before or after resection improves the results of surgery.

Palliative radiotherapy is on the other hand very suc-cessful in relieving distressing symptoms, particularly recur-rent haemoptysis, pain due to erosion of a rib and metastases in other bones. It is also often effective in easing the severe pain of apical tumours involving the brachial plexus and root pains associated with spinal metastases. Other indications are extensive invasion of the mediastinal lymph nodes with dyspnoea, dysphagia or obstruction of the superior vena cava.

Palliative

Cytotoxic drugs

These drugs, given alone or as adjuvants to surgery, do not pro-long life. Temporary remission often follows cyclophosphamide and other cytotoxic drugs, but all of them cause unpleasant side effects. They may be used as an alternative to radiotherapy for the relief of mediastinal obstruction.

The success of treatment with a combination of several cytotoxic drugs in other tumours revived interest in the ap-plication of these treatment schedules to carcinoma of the bronchus. Recent reports suggest that the simultaneous use of three or four cytotoxic drugs, with or without radiotherapy, is followed by temporary remission in small cell anaplastic car-cinoma of the bronchus. Even so, few patients survive for more than one year. The unpleasant effects of treatment should be set against this small gain.

It would be reasonable to hope that earlier diagnosis will improve the success of treatment. The results of 6 monthly routine X-rays of the chest have been disappointing. More in-tensive methods of early diagnosis by a combination of X-rays, sputum cytology and bronchoscopy are under trial, but it is clear that such time-consuming, expensive and sometimes unpleasant methods of investigation are not suitable for general use.

7 Pleural effusions

Aetiology – Investigations – Differential diagnosis – Tumours of the pleura – Complications – Treatment

Aetiology

Advances in the treatment of pulmonary infections are reflected by the lower incidence and changing aetiology of pleural effusions. Before the introduction of chemotherapy a serous effusion in young adults was regarded as evidence of a recent tuberculous infection. Pleurisy complicating untreated pneumonia often progressed to empyema requiring drainage. Cancer of the lung presenting with an effusion was less common than it is today.

At present most serous effusions are secondary to pyogenic respiratory infections sterilized by antibiotics. Tuberculous pleurisy is becoming increasingly rare so that effusions of rheumatoid or viral origin are more likely to be correctly diagnosed. The incidence of neoplastic effusions is increasing.

Exudates and transudates The customary distinction between inflammatory exudates and transudates, based on the colour, cytology and protein content of the fluid, is of little practical value. Effusions due to the transudation of fluid are readily diagnosed by their association with peripheral oedema, raised jugular venous pressure and other signs of heart failure. Transudates are often bilateral and small, seldom rising above the level of the 4th costal cartilage. They accumulate silently, while inflammatory exudates are usually preceded by pain and other symp-

119

toms of pleurisy. Most neoplastic effusions are painless, but they are usually much larger than transudates.

Investigations
Clinical signs

Percussion

Dull percussion note with absent breath and voice sounds over the base of the lung are reliable signs of a pleural effusion in a young patient with no previous history of respiratory disease. When the effusion complicates pneumonia or cancer these signs are more ambiguous. They may be due to solid lung beyond an obstructed bronchus, or fluid in the pleural cavity, or both.

Auscultation

Bronchial breathing, heard through compressed lung at the upper boundary of a large effusion, may be mistaken for a sign of pulmonary consolidation. Selective transmission of high frequencies lends a bleating quality to the voice sounds heard through a thin layer of fluid near the top of the effusion. This sign, known as aegophony, was valuable in the past, when a pleural effusion and solid lung had to be distinguished entirely by clinical signs. Friction between two roughened layers of the pleura alongside an effusion may generate adventitious sounds. These interrupted sounds are generally longer and lower pitched than crackling originating from the lung, but a pleural rub and pulmonary crackles may be indistinguishable.

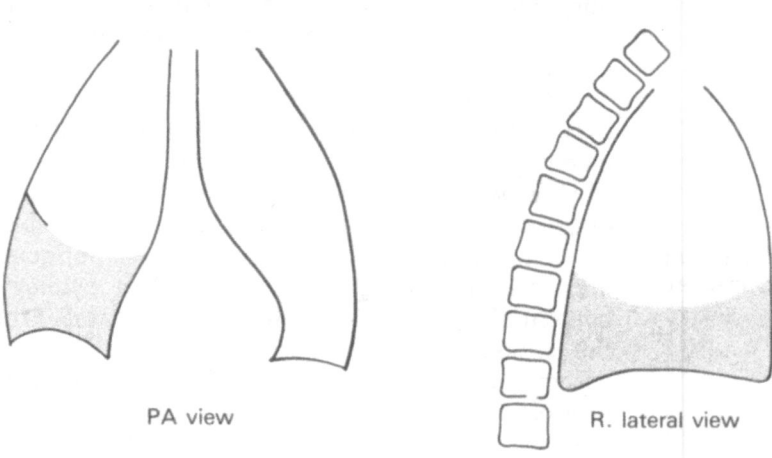

PA view   R. lateral view

R. Pleural effusion

Figure 7.1

X-rays

Few physicians have enough confidence in clinical signs to explore the chest with a needle until the effusion has been confirmed by an X-ray. A small effusion casts a dense shadow over the base of the lung, with a gradual transition through haziness into normal translucency. The upper limit of the fluid on the antero-posterior view is not clearly defined, except in the axillary line, where the rays strike the fluid tangentially. The impression that the fluid rises higher in the axilla than against the anterior and posterior chest wall is an optical illusion (Figure 7.1).

Small effusions filling the costophrenic angle may be missed when the lower lobe is airless. Encysted effusions lying against the posterior chest wall cast a well circumscribed, rounded shadow in the lateral projection, which may be mistaken for a tumour (Figure 7.2). Interlobar extension of the fluid is easily recognized, but an isolated interlobar effusion, persisting after the rest of the fluid has been absorbed, may be indistinguishable from segmental atelectasis.

Pleural thickening   Thickening or calcification of the parietal pleura in isolated patches (pleural plaques), or casting widespread bilateral dense shadows parallel with the ribs, is occasionally discovered in apparently healthy subjects. In the past they were attributed to healed caseous tuberculosis of the pleura. The usual cause of pleural plaques today is a symptomless chronic inflammatory reaction to asbestos. They are harmless, but are occasionally associated with a benign serous effusion.

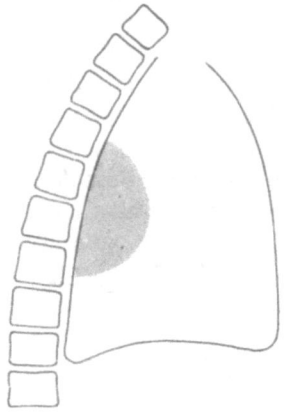

Posteriorly encysted effusion

Figure 7.2

The relation of plaques to malignant tumours of the pleura is uncertain.

Examination of the fluid

Aspiration

Aspiration of a small sample of fluid is the first step in the investigation of a pleural effusion. The needle should be introduced just below the upper limit of the dull percussion note posteriorly or in the axillary line. Lower down the two layers of the pleura may be fused, or a sediment of fibrin clots may obstruct the needle.

The chest wall is infiltrated with 5–10 ml 0.5% lignocaine, paying particular attention to the skin and the extrapleural tissues. A long needle, mounted on a 10 ml syringe, is then advanced gently into the pleural space, applying constant suction. A small sample of fluid (5–10 ml) is withdrawn and transferred into a glass or plastic container. This is a simple, painless procedure which can be safely performed in the consulting room or in the patient's home.

Colour

Pleural fluid is often described as straw coloured, although it may be any shade of yellow or orange. Effusions containing few cells are limpid or faintly turbid, while fluid with a high polymorph count is turbid, opaque or frankly purulent. Rare causes of turbidity are fat globules in chylous effusions, and cholesterol which produces a shimmering effect in some chronic encysted effusions. Blood staining is easily recognized. In small samples it is frequently due to the trauma of aspiration.

Chemistry

The protein content of the fluid is above 30 g/l in exudates and below this figure in transudates. These two varieties of effusion can be easily distinguished on other grour 's (p. 119). A very low glucose content (less than 1.1 mmol/l; 20 mg/100 ml) is one of the features of rheumatoid pleurisy.

Cytology

A report on the white cells in the fluid is of considerable diagnostic value. At the start of pyogenic infections all the cells are polymorphs. They are gradually replaced by lymphocytes when the fluid has been sterilized by antibiotics. Tuberculous effusions contain a mixture of polymorphs and lymphocytes at first, and become purely lymphocytic later on. Eosinophils in the fluid usually indicate a reaction to non-specific irritants, particularly blood in the pleural cavity. In some connective tissue diseases and in eosinophilic consolidation of the lung eosinophilia in pleural fluid is associated with a raised blood eosinophil count. If a tumour is suspected the fluid should be centrifuged, the sediment embedded in paraffin and examined for neoplastic cells.

Culture   The fluid should always be cultured for pyogenic organisms and tubercle bacilli. Pyogenic organisms are seldom isolated, because most effusions complicating pneumonia are sterilized by antibiotics. In tuberculous pleurisy, *M. tuberculosis* can be grown by special techniques from about 80% of effusions. In routine laboratory practice the yield of positive cultures from tuberculous effusions is less than 50%.

Biopsy

Skilful biopsy of the pleura with the Abrams biopsy punch is painless and safe. It is usually combined with diagnostic aspiration of fluid, but as the procedure requires the facilities of a minor operation it should be done in hospital. Only a small proportion of these minute tissue samples taken at random yields a firm histological diagnosis.

Biopsy specimens taken through the thoracoscope are more rewarding. The whole pleural cavity is inspected for miliary tubercles and neoplastic nodules, and a suitable specimen is removed under direct vision. The best method of all is a limited thoracotomy which seldom fails to produce conclusive histological evidence. For obvious reasons it should be reserved for cases where other diagnostic procedures have failed.

Differential diagnosis
Serous effusions

Pneumonia   The most common cause of a serous effusion is pleurisy complicating pneumonia. Widespread infection of the pleural cavity in untreated bacterial pneumonia is associated with a severe acute illness and a large purulent effusion. Acute pyogenic infections of the pleura are now either prevented, or aborted at an early stage by timely treatment with antibiotics. They are represented by sterile, symptomless effusions, discovered during or immediately after an acute lung infection.

The fluid is clear or faintly turbid. It contains predominantly polymorphs, which are gradually replaced by lymphocytes. The effusion does not reaccumulate after aspiration and usually disappears within a month.

Infarct   Serous effusion may also develop during non-bacterial (mycoplasmal or viral) pneumonia, and after pulmonary infarc-

123

tion. They are small and tend to be reabsorbed rapidly without treatment.

Tuberculous pleurisy

A common problem is the differential diagnosis between a tuberculous pleural effusion and a serous effusion complicating pneumonia. The usual history in both conditions is an acute pyrexial illness with cough and chest pain, treated at home with antibiotics. Some of these patients are admitted to hospital during the second week of the illness with pyrexia and a serous pleural effusion. Further treatment then depends on whether the acute illness was tuberculous pleurisy or a pyogenic infection sterilized with antibiotics.

The cytology of the fluid, a mixture of polymorphs and lymphocytes, is similar in pneumonic and tuberculous pleurisy. M. *tuberculosis* is seldom seen in smears of pleural fluid, and even if it is eventually grown in culture the report is not available in under 6–12 weeks.

In these circumstances a history of previous episodes of chest or shoulder pain is an important clue to the diagnosis. Such a history is reported by about 50% of patients with tuberculous pleurisy. The recurrent pain suggests one or more previous minor infections of the pleura from an underlying tuberculous lesion. The source of the infection may be a primary focus in the lung, or a tuberculous mediastinal lymph node, or more rarely a tuberculous abscess in the chest wall or dorsal spine.

The subsequent course of these two varieties of acute pleurisy is different. The fever in tuberculous pleurisy often continues for 4–6 weeks and the ESR remains high much longer than in pyogenic infections. The effusion is usually larger and is absorbed more slowly. Antituberculosis drugs have no immediate effect on the temperature, ESR, or on the rate of reabsorption of the fluid.

Tuberculous pleurisy is now uncommon in the native population of Western countries, but is still seen amongst young immigrants. In elderly men disseminated tuberculosis presenting with a pleural effusion or polyserositis may be mistaken for carcinomatosis.

Neoplastic effusions

A serous or blood-stained effusion may be the first sign of a disseminated tumour. The fluid accumulates silently and may remain undetected until it causes breathlessness. The primary tumour is often in the lung in men and in the breast in women. Other malignant tumours, especially carcinoma of the stomach and the ovary, may also metastasize to the pleura. Primary malignant tumours of the pleura are rare and unlike

Pleural effusions

secondary deposits they are painful. Malignant effusions reaccumulate after aspiration.

A sterile serous effusion in carcinoma of the bronchus does not necessarily mean that the tumour is inoperable. As in primary bacterial pneumonia, it may be due to a pyogenic infection of the pleura complicating bronchial obstruction, sterilized by antibiotics. Similarly a serous or blood-stained effusion following a pulmonary infarct in a patient with lung cancer should not be diagnosed as carcinomatosis of the pleura without further proof.

Meigs' syndrome is a benign ovarian tumour accompanied by ascites and a pleural effusion, which disappear when the tumour is removed. The pleural effusion is attributed to leakage of ascitic fluid into the chest through a congenital defect in the diaphragm with a pinhole communication between the peritoneal and pleural cavities.

Rheumatoid arthritis is occasionally associated with a serous pleural effusion, developing simultaneously with inflammations of the small joints of the hands. In others the effusion precedes the polyarthritis by several weeks or months.

Rheumatoid effusions are small or of moderate size, containing scanty lymphocytes or polymorphs. Other features which may help with the diagnosis are a low glucose content of the pleural fluid (less than 1.1 mmol/l; 20 mg/100 ml), rheumatoid factor in the serum, and rheumatoid nodules seen through the thoracoscope.

The fluid tends to reaccumulate after aspiration for several months, but eventually clears up, often leaving the pleura thickened.

None of these features is constant, so that a firm diagnosis may not be possible until it is confirmed by other clinical manifestations of rheumatoid arthritis.

Pleurisy with serous effusion may be one of the manifestations of systemic lupus erythematosus. It is frequently bilateral and may be accompanied by pericarditis. The fluid contains mononuclear cells and sometimes LE cells. The diagnosis rests on serological tests and association with other clinical signs of the disease.

A collection of pus under the diaphragm may be accompanied by a serous pleural effusion containing a mixture of polymorphs and lymphocytes. If the abscess is not drained, the infection may spread to the pleura and the effusion becomes purulent.

There is seldom any difficulty in recognizing the cause of

Meigs' syndrome

Rheumatoid pleurisy

SLE

Subphrenic abscess

Transudates

125

these effusions. They are nearly always due to heart failure with peripheral oedema. Less common causes are nephrosis, and hepatic failure with hypoproteinaemia. Bilateral pleural transudates may also develop in constrictive pericarditis.

Purulent effusions

Empyema is now uncommon because bacterial infections of the lung are treated early and intensively with antibiotics. Even so, a collection of pus, encysted over the posterior surface of the lower lobe, may be mistaken for pneumonia or a lung abscess.

Exploration of the pleura with a needle of suitable length and calibre is an essential investigation in all patients who remain pyrexial after an acute respiratory infection, with a raised white cell count and clubbing of the fingers. In these circumstances any residual shadow lying close to the chest wall should be regarded as an empyema, until this has been excluded by thorough, and if necessary repeated, exploration of the chest with an aspirating needle.

Haemorrhagic effusions

Blood-stained fluid

A serous effusion may be contaminated with blood if a large vessel in the chest wall is punctured. In small samples this may be misinterpreted as general blood-staining of the fluid. Haemorrhagic effusions are common in malignant tumours infiltrating the pleura. They may accompany pulmonary infarction and also occur occasionally in tuberculous pleurisy.

Haemothorax

Heavily blood-stained fluid is indistinguishable with the naked eye from haemothorax, where bleeding into the pleural cavity is followed by exudation of serous fluid. Dilution of a haemothorax, however, seldom reduces the haemoglobin concentration to less than 7 g/100 ml, while haemorrhagic exudates contain less than 2 g/100 ml. The source of the bleeding is often an obvious injury. When a vascular adhesion is torn in spontaneous pneumothorax the pleural cavity contains air as well as blood.

Tumours of the pleura
Localized mesothelioma (fibroma)

This is a rare tumour, usually discovered by routine radiography. Its clinical importance lies in the fact that it is sometimes associated with clubbing of the fingers and osteoarthropathy with severe wrist and ankle pains. Resection of the tumour promptly relieves these symptoms.

126

Table 7.1 Pleural effusions

Diagnosis	Size and appearance	Cytology*	Clinical features
Postpneumonic	Small, clear turbid or purulent	P or P + L	Pain, fever, productive cough
Pulmonary infarct	Small, clear or blood-stained	L or L + RC	Pain, blood-stained sputum
Tuberculous	Medium or large, clear	L or L + P	Recent and *previous* chest pain
Neoplastic	Large, clear or blood-stained	Scanty L, neoplastic cells	Dyspnoea or silent
Rheumatoid	Small or medium, clear	L	Joint pains or silent
SLE	Medium (bilateral), clear	L LE cells	Chest pain, other signs of SLE
Subphrenic abscess	Small, clear, turbid or purulent	P	History of abdominal emergency
Transudates	Small, clear	Mesothelial cells	Heart failure, nephrosis, constrictive pericarditis
Haemothorax	Small or medium, heavily blood-stained	RC	Trauma, spontaneous pneumothorax

* (P: polymorphs)
 (L: lymphocytes)
 (RC: red cells)

Diffuse malignant mesothelioma

Although it has been known for a long time that inhalation of asbestos dust may cause pulmonary fibrosis, the association with malignant mesothelioma of the pleura was recognized only in recent years. Small amounts of asbestos dust, inhaled during casual exposure, are sufficient to sow the seeds of these pleural tumours. The delay between exposure and the first sign of a mesothelioma may be as long as 40 years. The tumour gradually extends over the surface of the lung as well as in the parietal pleura, infiltrating the interlobar fissures, pericardium and the chest wall.

Pain is an early symptom. It helps to distinguish mesotheliomata from metastatic tumours of the pleura, which are usually painless. The pleural cavity fills with a serous or blood-stained effusion, which tends to recur in spite of repeated aspiration, and is replaced later by solid tumour.

Pathologists frequently disagree about the histological diagnosis of these tumours, because a common variety of mesothelioma resembles adenocarcinoma of the lung. A precise diagnosis is important, since patients with mesotheliomata, unlike those with cancer of the lung, qualify for industrial injuries benefit.

Complications

Most serous effusions are reabsorbed, leaving no trace, or at most obliteration of the costophrenic gutter. Persistent thickening of the pleura may follow tuberculous and rheumatoid effusions. The thickening often amounts to no more than a plaque of fibrosis which does not interfere with respiration.

Constrictive pleurisy

Extensive pleural fibrosis occurs in less than 1% of tuberculous effusions. The lung is encased in a rigid carapace of fibrous tissue, extending over the whole of the thoracic cage including the diaphragm. Ventilation and perfusion of the immobilized lung is then greatly reduced. The loss of function is severe, though it is sometimes reversible by excision of the pleura.

Amyloidosis

Chronic pyogenic infections of the pleura are now rare while tuberculous empyema has virtually disappeared since the end of artificial pneumothorax treatment. Secondary amyloidosis, formerly a dreaded complication of chronic empyema, has become a clinical curiosity. For the same reason empyema communicating with a bronchopleural fistula is now very uncommon, except as a complication of pneumonectomy.

Treatment
Postpneumonic effusions

Pleural effusions complicating non-bacterial (mycoplasmal, viral, etc.) pneumonia are small and are reabsorbed spontaneously. Bacterial infections of the lung are treated with antibiotics, so that the effusion is nearly always sterile by the time it is discovered. In such cases no treatment is necessary, other than optional aspiration of a few ounces of fluid at the time of the diagnostic paracentesis. If the fluid is purulent, turbid, or contains many pus cells, it is advisable to treat it as potentially infected even if the culture is sterile. Treatment with the appropriate antibiotic is essential if pyogenic organisms are cultured from the fluid.

Antibiotics

The objectives of treatment are sterilization of the fluid and re-expansion of the lung before the pleura is thickened by fibrin deposits and subsequent fibrosis. If the infecting organism can be isolated, the choice of antibiotic is determined

128

by its drug sensitivity. Otherwise ampicillin 1 g or amoxycillin 0.75 g, by mouth daily is the best choice for initial treatment. It should be supplemented by intrapleural injections of ampicillin 250 mg, or benzylpenicillin 300 mg (0.5 mega units), dissolved in 20 ml water at the end of each aspiration.

Therapeutic aspiration should be performed with a needle or an intravenous catheter attached to a 20 ml syringe, fitted with a three way tap. The purpose of aspiration is to expand the lung before it is fixed at a deflated volume by thickened pleura. As a general rule the chest should be aspirated dry twice a week, but if the patient complains of tightness in the chest, withdrawal of fluid must be stopped immediately.

Pleural effusions due to infection by pyogenic organisms almost always clear up under this treatment. Persistent pockets of fluid surrounded by thick pleura are now uncommon. Treatment with antibiotics by mouth and intrapleural injection, combined with repeated aspiration, is often effective even in such chronic effusions.

Surgical treatment
Open drainage or excision of the pleura is the last resort in chronic empyema that cannot be sterilized with antibiotics. Excision of the pleura may also be considered when a sterile effusion surrounded by thick pleura, or widespread constrictive pleurisy, seriously interferes with function of the lung.

Tuberculous pleurisy

Tuberculous pleural effusions are always associated with other obvious or latent lesions which may be disseminated or confined to the lung. Before the discovery of antituberculosis drugs the effusion usually reabsorbed without treatment, leaving no residual thickening of the pleura. Other tuberculous lesions appeared within a year in about 25% of patients.

Chemo-therapy
Antituberculosis drugs do not shorten the acute pyrexial stage of tuberculous pleurisy and do not hasten the reabsorption of fluid. They are very effective in preventing further manifestations of tuberculosis.

The aim of treatment, as in any other tuberculous infection, is the destruction of all tubercle bacilli. The dosage and length of treatment is identical with that in pulmonary tuberculosis: rifampicin and isoniazid for 9 months, supplemented with ethambutol during the first 2 months (Table 5.2).

Aspiration
Therapeutic aspiration is unnecessary if the effusion is small or of moderate size. Large effusions should be reduced in size until the patient is comfortable. Nothing is to be

gained from an attempt at complete evacuation of the fluid. It does not hasten reabsorption and does not improve the prospects of good functional recovery. Respiratory movements of the chest and diaphragm nearly always return to normal, even when the fluid has persisted for several months.

Cortico-
steroids

Corticosteroids shorten the acute stage of tuberculous pleurisy. The temperature returns to normal earlier and the fluid is reabsorbed more rapidly. Prednisone 15 mg by mouth daily for 2 weeks may be given to acutely ill patients or to those with large effusions. Apart from this immediate palliative effect there is no long-term advantage in treating tuberculous pleurisy with corticosteroids.

Neoplastic effusions

Malignant tumours of the pleura, whether primary or secondary, cannot be eradicated. All that treatment can achieve is to relieve pain and dyspnoea and to prevent or delay reaccumulation of fluid.

Severe pain is unusual in pleural metastases but common in diffuse mesothelioma infiltrating the chest wall. Radiotherapy and cytotoxic drugs are ineffective against this tumour, while surgical intervention may actually accelerate infiltration of the chest wall. Even aspiration of fluid may be followed by spread of the mesothelioma along the needle track. In these circumstances it is best to avoid all local treat-

Analgesics ment. The pain can sometimes be controlled with anti-inflammatory drugs (phenylbutazone or indomethacin) or with potent analgesics. For intractable pain chordotomy is justifiable in the last resort.

In large effusions, carcinomatosis of the pleura associated with dyspnoea can be relieved, at least temporarily, by aspiration of the fluid. When frequently repeated aspirations become intolerable an attempt should be made to obliterate the pleural cavity. This can be achieved by injecting a cytotoxic drug (thiotepa 45 mg, or mustine 20 mg in 10 ml saline) immediately after a complete aspiration. These drugs may destroy some neoplastic cells, but like other irritants they act mainly by inflaming the pleura and promoting fusion of its two layers.

Hormonal
treatment

Pleural metastases of carcinoma of the breast can sometimes be controlled for a time with corticosteroids, sex hormones or pituitary ablation. Effusions in disseminated carcinoma of the prostate may respond to castration and the administration of oestrogens.

130

Recurrent respiratory illness in children

Viral infections − Cystic fibrosis − Immune deficiencies −
Bronchiectasis

Viral infections

Immunity to viral respiratory infections is acquired gradually during childhood. There is a large variety of pathogenic viruses and the process of immunization involves many infections. Some of these are silent, others are accompanied by symptoms ranging in severity from a trivial cold to airway obstruction.

Age incidence These illnesses begin in infancy and their incidence reaches its peak at the age of 5 years when the child enters school. This is followed by a rapid decline, so that by the age of 8 the incidence is similar to that in the adult population.

Catarrhal Some children, usually referred to as 'catarrhal', are much
children more prone to respiratory illnesses than others. Whether their vulnerability is due to an immunological defect or to allergy is not known. Many children who become wheezy during each infection show other evidence of bronchial lability. They also wheeze after strenuous exercise and after inhalation of common allergens. Hypersensitivity to allergens is often demonstrable by skin tests, eosinophilia, and a high IgE titre in the serum.

Asthma Whether these episodes of wheezing should be called asthma is a matter of definition. There is no sharp dividing line between children who wheeze only during respiratory infections and others who are prone to short attacks of dyspnoea

131

and wheezing at other times as well. What matters for practical purposes is that most of them recover by the age of 8 years.

Viruses   Severe pulmonary infections in young children are often due to the respiratory syncytial or parainfluenza viruses. In upper respiratory infections and in older children influenza, rhino-, adeno-, and enteroviruses are also common. These organisms can be identified by laboratory tests, but there is considerable overlap in their clinical manifestations.

Symptoms and signs

The usual upper respiratory symptoms are coryza, nasal obstruction, earache and sore throat. If the infection involves the lungs, the symptoms range from a mild cough to severe airway obstruction.

Airway obstruction   Most viral infections in children are minor illnesses. Respiratory obstruction at the epiglottis, larynx, or in the small airways may however develop with alarming speed and transform a trivial cold into a potentially fatal illness. Signs common to all these varieties of airway obstruction are dyspnoea, inspiratory recession of the ribs and cyanosis. Prostration and pallor are late signs of impending asphyxia and circulatory collapse. Wheezes and crackles indicate widespread narrowing of the intrathoracic airways.

Treatment

Antibiotics   Antibiotics are ineffective in viral infections and should not be prescribed merely to prevent secondary infections. Bacterial sinusitis and otitis media are uncommon complications in any event, and timely treatment with antibiotics brings them rapidly under control. These complications usually begin during the second week of the illness, with recurrence of pyrexia, accompanied by purulent nasal discharge, earache and a red, bulging eardrum.

Airway obstruction   Airway obstruction must be treated in hospital, where an oxygen tent, nebulizers, suction apparatus and facilities for intubation or tracheostomy are available. Bronchodilator drugs are ineffective in children under 2 years of age. Widespread airway obstruction in this age group is usually due to mucosal swelling and retained bronchial secretions. It often responds to humidification of the air with steam or a nebulizer. At this age viral and bacterial infections cannot be distinguished from allergic bronchial obstruction. It is best to play safe and to treat widespread airflow obstruction in young children with antibiotics.

In children over the age of 2 years bronchodilator drugs help to relieve dyspnoea and wheezing during infective episodes. Intal may be effective in preventing wheeziness, particularly when it is not confined to infections but is also provoked by exercise, emotional stress and inhaled allergens. The other symptoms of recurrent pyrexial illnesses in catarrhal children cannot be prevented by Intal, antibiotics or any other treatment.

Tonsillectomy

Many parents and some doctors believe in tonsillectomy, although there is no evidence that it reduces the number or severity of respiratory illnesses in catarrhal children. No other unnecessary operation is performed on a comparable scale.

In chronic respiratory obstruction by gross hypertrophy of nasopharyngeal lymphatic tissue removal of the tonsils and adenoids is justifiable. It is also possible that tonsillectomy prevents frequently recurring throat infections by pyogenic organisms. Such infections must not be confused with viral sore throats or with 'chronic tonsillitis', diagnosed by the usual unreliable criteria. Apart from these exceptions the operation should never be advised for recurrent respiratory illnesses in children.

Advice to parents

The management of these children requires much skill and patience. Most parents fear that the seemingly endless succession of nasal catarrh, sore throat, earache and bronchitis will permanently damage the child's health. They should be reassured that the child is likely to be well by the age of 8 and that there will be no residual disability.

It is more difficult to answer the question whether a child with frequently recurring short pyrexial respiratory illnesses, accompanied by wheezing, has asthma. An affirmative answer should always be qualified by an explanation that asthma includes many respiratory diseases, and that the outlook is particularly good when wheezing is confined to febrile respiratory infections. Complete recovery is the rule long before adolescence.

Cystic fibrosis

This is an hereditary abnormality of mucus secreting and other exocrine glands. Its earliest respiratory manifestation is a recurrent cough in infancy, followed by increasingly frequent

133

episodes of purulent bronchitis and sinusitis. These recurrent infections damage the bronchial wall and lead to bronchiectasis with persistent cough and purulent sputum.

Other symptoms of the disease include intestinal obstruction by impacted meconium at birth and steatorrhoea due to deficient pancreatic secretion. A reliable and painless screening test is estimation of sodium in sweat collected after pilocarpine iontophoresis. In children with cystic fibrosis the concentration of sodium is abnormally high (above 70 mmol/l).

When cystic fibrosis was first described over 40 years ago it was usually fatal during childhood. Now that severe pulmonary infections can be effectively treated, many survive into adult life.

These infections, which are often staphylococcal, must be treated early with the appropriate antibiotics. Postural drainage is helpful, as in other varieties of bronchiectasis. The effectiveness of humidification of the air in steam tents or with nebulizers is doubtful.

Immune deficiencies

Congenital defects of antibody production or cell-mediated immunity as a cause of recurrent respiratory infections in children and adults are uncommon. Many new syndromes have been described in recent years. Some of these are easily recognized by simple estimation of circulating antibodies. Others require elaborate investigations in special departments. The difficulty lies in selecting those children who might benefit from these time-consuming studies.

Bronchiectasis

The control of infectious fevers and tuberculosis, effective treatment of severe lung infections, and routine removal of inhaled foreign bodies led to a sharp fall in the prevalence of bronchiectasis in children. It still occurs sporadically as a congenital defect, and in association with immune deficiencies or cystic fibrosis.

The dilated bronchi may be visible on a plain X-ray. In others the persistence of clinical signs in the damaged lobe, or association with other congenital abnormalities (e.g. dextrocardia), draws attention to the possibility of bronchiectasis. Bronchography is not justifiable unless bronchiectasis confined to one lobe is suspected and resection is likely to be successful.

Fibrosing alveolitis

Diagnosis – Treatment

Definition The term 'alveolitis' was introduced in order to distinguish a group of relatively rare pulmonary diseases, characterized by cellular inflitration of the alveolar wall, from the more common pneumonias in which the alveoli fill with inflammatory exudate, but their walls remain intact. Unlike pneumonia, which usually resolves completely, alveolitis often leads to widespread pulmonary fibrosis.

Aetiology Fibrosing alveolitis includes diseases with similar clinical, radiological and functional features due to a variety of agents. Some of these are hypersensitivity reactions to inhaled allergens or to drugs. Others are associated with systemic connective tissue diseases. In the majority of cases the aetiology remains unknown.

Diagnosis

Fibrosing alveolitis is easily recognized once its possibility has been considered. Early diagnosis is important because disabling or fatal lung damage can sometimes be prevented by timely action.

Symptoms and signs The onset may be acute, with fever, cough, breathlessness and basal crackles, resembling a respiratory infection. The correct diagnosis is first suspected when there is no response to antibiotics. The dyspnoea and unproductive cough get progressively worse, although in cases where occasional inhala-

135

tion of an allergen is responsible there may be long remissions.

The timing of the basal crackles is characteristic. They are confined to inspiration and become more profuse as the lung approaches full inflation. They often become scanty and may be silenced altogether when the patient bends forward. Clubbing of the fingers and cyanosis are signs of more advanced disease.

X-rays

The X-rays in fibrosing alveolitis of obscure aetiology show stippling, starting in the lower zones and rising higher as the disease advances. In allergic alveolitis the micronodules often merge into large confluent opacities resembling consolidation, which may resolve, to be replaced by similar shadows in other parts of the lung. The later stages are similar in all varieties of fibrosing alveolitis. The shadows become confluent and are gradually replaced by a network of fibrous tissue interlaced between overdistended alveoli, forming a honeycomb pattern.

Pulmonary function

The functional damage consists of reduced distensibility of the lung and impaired gas exchange. The pulmonary compliance decreases progressively and the total lung capacity and vital capacity fall correspondingly lower. The carbon monoxide transfer is reduced while the arterial oxygen tension is still normal. Later on there is hypoxia during exertion and eventually at rest as well.

Allergic alveolitis

Farmer's lung

Farmer's lung, a combination of allergic bronchitis and alveolitis, due to the inhalation of antigens in mouldy hay, was first recognized over 50 years ago. More recently several other antigens, mostly fungal spores, have been identified in sporadic cases of allergic alveolitis. Most of these are occupational diseases seldom seen in general practice.

Bird fancier's lung

An important exception is bird fancier's lung, a potentially fatal variety of allergic alveolitis, due to the inhalation of antigens in the droppings of pigeons and budgerigars. These birds are harmless to most people, but some become sensitized by avian antigens and develop recurrent pyrexial episodes with headache, malaise, cough and breathlessness. At first these symptoms are often mistaken for mild respiratory infections. The lungs may be irreversibly damaged by the time the true cause of the disease is recognized.

The diagnosis rests on the clinical signs, X-ray appearances and lung function tests already described. It is confirmed by the demonstration of precipitins to avian serum proteins in the patient's blood. All further contact with the birds must then be avoided. Admission to hospital is advisable while the home is thoroughly cleaned of the dry dust of budgerigar droppings.

Treatment

Prednisone 30 mg daily is effective in allergic alveolitis and should be given while improvement, as judged by X-rays and respiratory function tests, continues. In other varieties of fibrosing alveolitis response to corticosteroids is less predictable. If there is no improvement in the X-ray appearances and respiratory function tests after 6 weeks on prednisone 30 mg daily, the treatment may be discontinued.

10 Spontaneous pneumothorax

Pathogenesis – Symptoms and Signs – Treatment

Pathogenesis

Bullae

Spontaneous pneumothorax, as seen in general practice, is nearly always the result of rupture of a bulla. If the bulla lies on the surface of the lung, air leaks directly into the pleural cavity. If it is buried in the depth of the lung, the air tracks along the peribronchial and perivascular connective tissue sheaths to the surface of the lung, where it raises subpleural blebs. Their rupture opens a path to the entry of air into the pleural cavity.

Tall stature

In healthy young adults the site of the air leak is usually a pleural tear over a previously silent bulla. The rest of the lung is normal and these patients do not develop emphysema later in life. The aetiology of the bullae is obscure. They are more common in tall thin young men, and it is possible that mechanical stresses associated with such a stature damage the apex of the

Emphysema

lung. When spontaneous pneumothorax occurs as a complication of asthma, chronic bronchitis or emphysema, widespread bullae are often visible on the chest X-ray.

Pleural pressure

Air continues to flow into the pleural cavity until the tear is sealed or until the intrapleural pressure is above atmospheric pressure throughout the respiratory cycle. In some cases, where the communication between the lung and the pleural cavity acts like a non-return valve, large amounts of air accumulate, displacing the mediastinum and interfering with ventilation of the opposite lung. Tension pneumothorax means

139

simply a large volume of gas in the pleural cavity with mediastinal displacement and respiratory distress.

Absorption The gases in the pleural cavity are slowly absorbed by diffusion into the capillary circulation. If the pleural tear is sealed and the lung remains normally distensible all gas is eventually reabsorbed. The communication may however reopen at any stage of re-expansion, letting more air into the pleural cavity.

Recurrence Inflammation of the pleura is rare in pneumothorax due to rupture of a bulla. The pleural cavity remains dry and the two layers of the pleura do not become adherent when the lung comes into contact with the chest wall. In these circumstances the pneumothorax may recur if the bulla ruptures again.

Symptoms and signs

In previously healthy subjects a symptomless pneumothorax may be discovered by a routine X-ray. More often it is accompanied by chest pain and breathlessness. If the pneumothorax is shallow these symptoms clear up within a day or two, long before the lung is fully re-expanded. In asthma and in elderly patients with widespread airflow obstruction pneumothorax is a serious additional handicap, accompanied by sudden increase of dyspnoea.

Unilateral absence of breath and voice sounds with a normal percussion note are reliable signs of air in the pleural cavity. Apart from pneumothorax this combination of clinical signs occurs only in unilateral emphysema or a large diaphragmatic hernia. Additional signs in a large pneumothorax are displacement of the mediastinum, rapid deep breathing, tachycardia and cyanosis.

Treatment

Healthy young adults with a shallow pneumothorax need no treatment. The chest should be X-rayed at weekly intervals until the lung has fully re-expanded. A large pneumothorax, or relapse during re-expansion, should be treated in hospital. A self-retaining catheter is introduced into the pleural cavity under local anaesthesia and connected with an underwater seal. Correct placement of the catheter is indicated by air bubbles escaping during expiration, and subatmospheric pleural pressure, shown by rise of the level of water in the tubing during inspiration.

The drainage tube is disconnected and clamped as soon as the bubbling ceases during tidal breathing. If a chest X-ray 24 hours later shows that the amount of gas in the pleura is not increasing, the catheter may be removed and further re-expansion can be left to nature.

Spontaneous pneumothorax complicating asthma, chronic bronchitis or emphysema should always be treated in hospital, so that a catheter can be introduced at the first sign of respiratory distress. The management of these patients is identical with that of previously healthy young adults, but their progress is less satisfactory, because the air leak often recurs during re-expansion of the lung.

Pleurodesis   Pleurodesis or thoracotomy is the next step if the pleural tear does not close, or reopens during re-expansion of the lung. This is recognized by persistent bubbling from the drainage tube and confirmed by measurement of the pleural pressure. The pleural cavity should then be inspected through a thoracoscope before deciding whether resection of the bulla, combined with surgical pleurodesis, is necessary. Alternatively obliteration of the pleural space by intrapleural injection of a chemical irritant may be sufficient.

Pleurodesis may also be advised to prevent recurrence of the pneumothorax. In healthy young adults the first two episodes are usually treated conservatively and pleurodesis is recommended only if the pneumothorax recurs again. In emphysematous patients the risks are much greater and the pleural space should be obliterated without waiting for a recurrence.

11 Pulmonary sarcoidosis

Natural history – Treatment

A common problem in sarcoidosis is whether the disease should be treated with corticosteroids or be allowed to run its natural course. Hypercalcaemia with the attendant risk of renal failure, and uveitis endangering the eyesight are generally accepted indications of treatment. Disfiguring cutaneous lesions are also often treated.

The decision is more difficult in pulmonary sarcoidosis which usually heals without treatment, leaving the lungs undamaged or lightly scarred, but occasionally ends in severe fibrosis and respiratory failure.

Natural history

Recovery Many apparently healthy patients with sarcoidosis first come under observation as a result of a routine X-ray which shows bilateral enlargement of the hilar lymph nodes. In 80% of these the X-ray appearances return to normal within a year. The outlook is even more favourable when the onset of hilar lymphadenopathy is accompanied by erythema nodosum.

In the remaining 20%, disseminated mottling appears in the lungs, usually without any symptom of pulmonary disease. The prognosis is still very good. Complete resolution takes place within 2 years in 80% of this group. Even when some abnormal shadows persist, pulmonary function remains normal.

Deterioration In 5% of all patients under observation the shadows increase in density and invade previously intact territories of the lung. Deterioration may be continuous or interrupted by periods of stability. At this stage most patients complain of dyspnoea on exertion and an unproductive cough. Arrest of the disease and partial resolution is still possible. In others the granulomata are replaced by scars, recognized by a change from stippling to linear shadows and overdistension of the intervening alveoli. Extensive pulmonary fibrosis leads to severe breathlessness, respiratory failure and eventually death from hypoxia or pulmonary hypertension.

The early stages of this progression from hilar adenopathy to pulmonary infiltration and fibrosis may pass unnoticed in patients who come under observation complaining of dyspnoea or some extrapulmonary manifestation of sarcoidosis. The prognosis is then less favourable, although the condition of the lungs may still remain stable or improve without treatment.

Bronchial stenosis An uncommon presentation of pulmonary sarcoidosis is dyspnoea with wheezing, due to intrabronchial sarcoid granulomata. Bronchial obstruction or stenosis by these small lesions causes disproportionately severe damage and requires early treatment.

Treatment

Immediate effects Corticosteroids are immediately effective at all stages of pulmonary sarcoidosis, short of fibrosis. There is striking improvement in the X-ray appearances, symptoms, and pulmonary function, which is usually maintained as long as treatment with adequate doses is continued. Termination of treatment or abrupt reduction of the dose is often followed by prompt clinical, radiological and functional deterioration.

Long term effects It is possible that corticosteroids merely suppress the manifestations of sarcoidosis, without any long term advantage, so that the ultimate outcome in treated and untreated patients is identical. If this could be shown to be true, the long term use of corticosteroids, with its well known complications, would not be justified. A controlled study of the long term progress of sarcoidosis, with random allocation of corticosteroid treatment, has never been carried out, for ethical reasons. In these circumstances it is reasonable to take the view that corticosteroids not only delay pulmonary fibrosis, but may prevent it altogether if continued until the disease is no longer active.

Indications With the exception of erythema nodosum and polyarthritis at the beginning of the illness, when prednisone may be given for 2−3 weeks to relieve pain, a decision to treat sarcoidosis commits the patient to several years on corticosteroids. The right strategy in a disease with a generally favourable prognosis is to withhold treatment while spontaneous recovery is still possible, but not to delay until irreversible pulmonary fibrosis is already established. This difficult decision should not be taken until a period of observation has confirmed progressive deterioration of the X-rays and pulmonary function. Bronchial stenosis due to sarcoid granuloma in a major bronchus should be treated as soon as possible.

The earliest stages of fibrosis cannot be recognized on the chest X-ray. By the time the linear shadows of scarring and overdistension of the intervening lung tissue are obvious, the fibrosis is irreversible. It is therefore usual to accept a progressive increase in the extent and density of the shadows as an indication for treatment, but only if the deterioration is confirmed by pulmonary function tests. For this purpose serial measurements of the total lung capacity, vital capacity, carbon monoxide transfer, and pulmonary compliance are the most useful tests.

Dosage The initial dose of prednisone is 30 mg daily. After 6 weeks the dose is reduced by steps of 5 mg at monthly intervals. A maintenance dose of 10 mg daily is often sufficient to stabilize the X-ray appearances and respiratory measurements, without causing unwanted effects.

Duration After a year's treatment the dose should be tentatively reduced by 2.5 mg at monthly intervals. If the X-rays or breathing tests deteriorate, the usual maintenance dose is restored for another 12 months. The condition of most patients remains stable on this regime. Treatment should be continued indefinitely or until the annual trial reduction of the dose shows that the disease is no longer active.

Further reading

1. *Asthma*. Clark, T. J. H. and Godfrey, S. (1977) (London: Chapman and Hall)
2. *Immunology of the Lung*. Turner-Warwick, M. (1978) (London: Edward Arnold)
3. *Lung Sounds*. Forgacs, P. (1978) (London: Baillière Tindall)
4. *Modern Drug Treatment of Tuberculosis*. 5th Edn. Ross, J. D. and Horne, N. W. (1978) (London: Chest, Heart and Stroke Association)
5. *Principles of Chest X-ray Diagnosis*. 4th Edn. Simon, S. (1978) (Butterworth)
6. *Pulmonary Pathophysiology – the Essentials*. West, J. B. (1977) (Oxford: Blackwell Scientific Publications)
7. *Respiratory Diseases*. 2nd Edn. Crofton, J. and Douglas, A. (1975) (Oxford: Blackwell Scientific Publications)
8. *Respiratory Illness in Children*. Williams, H. E. and Phelan, P. D. (1975) (Oxford: Blackwell Scientific Publications)
9. *Respiratory Physiology – the Essentials*. 2nd Edn. West, J. B. (1979) (Oxford: Blackwell Scientific Publications)
10. *Smoking or Health*. Royal College of Physicians, 3rd Report (1977) (Tunbridge Wells: Pitman Medical)

Index

abscess
  lung 13, 30, 39
  subphrenic 14, 47, 125
abscess-like appearance of lung
    cancer 112
achalasia of the cardia, and
    recurrent pneumonia 45
acid fast bacilli 94–95
adenoids, removal 133
adenovirus
  and pneumonia 37
  in children 132
adrenaline *see* bronchodilators
aegophony 25, 120
airflow obstruction 55, 56 Fig. 3.2
  see also named diseases
airway obstruction in children
    children, treatment 132–133
allergens
  avoidance 84–85
  and fibrosing alveolitis 136
  hyposensitization 83–84
allergic alveolitis 136–137
  treatment 137
allergic bronchitis
  cough 11
  eosinophils in sputum 57
allergy
  in asthma 70, 71
  in catarrhal children 131
  see also allergens
alveolar cell tumour 106
  see also cancer of the lung

alveolitis, description 135
  see also fibrosing alveolitis
aminophyllin, in treatment of asthma
    80, 85
amoxycillin 62, 129
ampicillin 50, 62, 129
amyloidosis 128
anaemia, dyspnoea in 19
anaerobes 13, 37, 40
analgesics
  in treating lung infections 52
  in treating neoplastic effusions
    130
anaplastic tumours 106
  see also cancer of the lung
ankylosing spondylitis
  chronic respiratory failure in 39
  apical fibrosis in 93
antibodies
  in aspergillosis 15, 76
  in immune deficiencies 134
  in hypersensitivity reactions 74
antibiotics
  in chronic bronchitis 62
  in cystic fibrosis 134
  in lung infections 50–51, 132
  in pleural effusions 5, 128–129
  see also named antibiotics
antiinflammatory drugs, in
    mesothelioma 130
antituberculosis drugs 99–102
  reserve drugs 102
  in tuberculous pleurisy 129

149

asbestos
  and cancer of the lung 106
  and malignant mesothelioma 127
  pleural plaques 121
asbestosis 33
aspergillosis, allergic
    bronchopulmonary 76
  see also antibodies
Aspergillus fumigatus
  in healed tuberculous cavities 94
  and haemoptysis 15
  hypersensitivity in aspergillosis
    76
asphyxia
  and death in chronic bronchitis
    during infection 61, 67
aspirin, and asthma 70, 71
asthma
  in catarrhal children 131–132,
    133
  classification 71–72
  clinical features 72–73
  danger signals 73
  death in 70, 78, 85
  definition 69
  differential diagnosis 74–77
    Table 4.2
  dyspnoea 18
  exercise provocation 69, 73, 78
  expiratory flow rate in 32
  investigations
    respiratory measurements 73
    hypersensitivity tests 73–74
  monophonic wheeze 26 Fig. 1.6
  pathogenesis 69–71 Table 4.1
    allergy 70
    bronchial lability 69
    other factors 70–71
  pneumothorax in 139, 141
  polyphonic wheeze 27–28
  prognosis 77–78, 133
  treatment 86 Table 4.3
    allergen avoidance 84–85
    breathing exercises 84
    bronchodilators 78–80
    corticosteroids 81–83
    emergency treatment 85–86
    hyposensitization 83–84
    hypnoptherapy 84
    Intal 80–81
    psychotherapy 84
    sodium cromoglycate *see* Intal

atropine, *see* bronchodilators
avian proteins, precipitins to, in bird
    fancier's lung 137
barium meal, in investigating
    recurrent pneumonia 45
benign lung tumours 114
benzylpenicillin 50, 129,
    see also antibiotics
betamethasone, *see* corticosteroids
BCG vaccination 96, 97
bird fancier's lung 136–137
blood gases
  in asthma 73
  in chronic respiratory failure 60
  in fibrosing alveolitis 136
  see also PCO_2, PO_2
bovine cough 13
bromhexine, in treatment of chronic
    bronchitis 62
breath sounds 23–25
breathing exercises
  in asthma 84
  in chronic bronchitis 66
breathing patterns 16, 17 Fig. 1.2
breathing tests
  CO transfer 33
  in chronic bronchitis 54
  forced expiratory flow rate 32
    Fig. 1.12
  forced expiratory volume (FEV_1)
    32 Fig. 1.12, 33
  forced expiratory time 33
  peak expiratory flow rate (PEFR)
    33, 34 Table 1.1
  in pulmonary sarcoidosis 145
  regional lung function tests 34
breathlessness 16–21
  in chronic bronchitis 39, 54
  in fibrosing alveolitis 135
  in neoplastic effusion 124
  in pneumothorax 140
  in pulmonary sarcoidosis 144
'brittle' asthmatics 72, *see also*
    asthma
bronchial adenocarcinoma 106,
    see also cancer of the lung
bronchial adenoma 114
bronchial lability
  in asthma 69–70
  in catarrhal children 131
bronchial stenosis

and pulmonary sarcoidosis 144,
145
tuberculous 45
bronchiectasis
bronchography 134
in children 134
in chronic bronchitis 58
clubbing of fingers in 30, 44
in cystic fibrosis 134
and suppurative pneumonia 44
treatment 52, 58
bronchitis *see* chronic bronchitis
bronchoscopy
in lung cancer 112–113
bronchodilators
in asthma 72, 73, 78–80
in children 132–133
in chronic bronchitis 57, 62–64
dangers 78–79
inhalation technique 63, 79
and PEFR 33
by PPV 66
unwanted effects 63, 64
bronchography, in bronchiectasis
134
bronchopneumonia *see* pneumonia
bronchorrhoea 14
budgerigars and bird fancier's lung
136–137
bullae and pneumothorax 139, 140,
141

cancer of the lung
aetiology 105–106
classification 106
clinical signs 110
differential diagnosis 48, 114
endocrine syndromes 108–109
investigations
bronchoscopy 112–113
X-ray 111 Fig. 6.1, 112
mortality 105
neurological syndromes 108
pain in 22, 108, 118
presentation 106–110, 109
Table 6.1
prevention 114–117
progress 110, 112
smoking 114–117
symptoms 107–108
treatment
drugs 118

radiotherapy 114, 117, 118
surgery 117
Candida albicans, thrush and
corticosteroids aerosols 82
carbenicillin, in treatment of lung
infections 51
carcinogens 106
in tobacco smoke 116
carcinoma, alveolar cell 14
cat scratch disease mimicking
tuberculous adenitis 95
catarrhal children 74, 131–133
cephalosporins, in treatment of
pneumonia 50
chest pain *see* pain
Chlamydia psittaci see (psittacosis)
37, 40, 50
chronic bronchitis
breath sounds 24
clinical features
airflow obstruction 55
mucus secretion 55
cough 35
complications 59–60
crackles 28, 29 Fig. 1.9
differential diagnosis 58, 74
dyspnoea 16, 18
early manifestations 13
and heart failure 59
infective exacerbations 39
investigations
bronchodilator response 57
FEV_1 56–57
PEFR 56–57
sputum tests 57
X-ray 57
mortality 53 Fig. 3.1
pathology 53–54
pneumothorax 139, 141
prevalence 53
prevention 61, 114–117
recurrent pneumonia in 44, 45
summary 67 Table 3.1
treatment
antibiotics 62
bronchodilators 62–64
corticosteroids 64–65
Intal 64
oxygen 65–66
wheezes 26–28
chronic respiratory failure 39
in chronic bronchitis 39,

60–61
management   67–68
cigarette smoking *see* smoking
clinical signs
   auscultation
      breath sounds   23–25, 24
      Fig. 1.4, 25 Fig. 1.5
      wheezes (rhonchi)   25–28
      crackles (râles, crepitations)
      28–29, 28 Fig. 1.9, 29
      Fig. 1.10
      pleural sounds   30
   clubbing of fingers   30
   cyanosis   30
   percussion   23, 120
   pursed lip breathing   30–31
clubbing of fingers
   in cancer of the lung   110
   in chronic empyema   43
   diagnostic value   30
   in fibrosing alveolitis   136
   and lung abscess   40
   and mesothelioma   126
   and purulent pleural effusions
      126
coliform bacilli, significance in
      sputum   41
compulsive sighing   20
   differential diagnosis from asthma
      76
   spirogram   20 Fig. 1.3
congenital abnormalities and
      bronchiectasis   134
cordotomy, to relieve intractable
      pain   130
cor pulmonale in chronic bronchitis
      59
corticosteroids
   choice   83
   in treatment of
      asthma   72, 74, 81–83
      bronchonhoea   14
      chronic bronchitis   64–65
      fibrosing alveolitis   33, 137
      neoplastic effusions   130
      pulmonary sarcoidosis
143–145
      tuberculous pleurisy   130
costochondritis and chest pain   23
CO transfer   33
   in fibrosing alveolitis   136
   see also breathing tests

co-trimoxazole
   in treatment of chronic bronchitis
      62
   in treatment of pneumonia   50
cough   11
   in cancer of the lung   107
   in chronic bronchitis   55
   in fibrosing alveolitis   135
   impaired efficiency   36
   syncope   13
   varieties   12 Fig. 1.1
coughing, assisted, in treatment of
      chronic bronchitis   66
Coxiella burneti, see Q fever
crackles *see also* clinical signs
      28–30
   in chronic bronchitis   39, 55
   in fibrosing alveolitis   135, 136
   and pleural effusions   120
   and tuberculosis   90
   in viral infections of children   132
crepitations *see* crackles
Cushing syndrome, in lung cancer
      109
cyanosis   30
cyclophosphamide, in treatment of
      lung cancer   118
cystic fibrosis   35, 45, 133–134
cysts, and recurrent pneumonia   45
cytology of pleural fluid   122–123
cytology of sputum, in diagnosis of
      lung cancer   113, 118
cytotoxic drugs
   in cancer of the lung   118
   in carcinomatosis of the pleura
      130
   and mesothelioma   130

death
   in asthma   85
   from cancer of the lung   105, 112
   from pulmonary sarcoidosis   144
   and smoking   115
   from tuberculosis   87, 92
dexamethasone *see* corticosteroids
dextrocardia   134
diaphragmatic hernia   140
disseminated tuberculosis *see*
      tuberculosis
disodium cromoglycate *see* Intal
drugs *see also* antibiotics,
      bronchodilators, corticosteroids
      etc.

causing asthma   70-71
for treating asthma   86 Table 4.3
dynamic compression of bronchi
   31 Fig. 1.11, 32
dysphagia, in lung cancer   108, 112,
   118
dyspnoea *see* breathlessness

effort syndrome   19
effusions *see* pleural effusions
emphysema
   breath sounds in   24, 25 Fig. 1.5
   bronchodilator response   57
   and chronic bronchitis   54, 55, 59
   definition   59
   dynamic compression of bronchi in
      31 Fig. 1.11
   dyspnoea in   18
   expiratory flow rate in   32
   and pneumothorax   139, 140, 141
   wheeze in   28
empyema   14, 126
   clubbing in   30
   complicating pneumonia   43, 126,
      128
   surgery in   129
   treatment   44, 128-129
endocrine syndromes, associated
      with lung cancer   108
enterovirus, in children   132
eosinophils
   in aspergillosis   76
   significance in pleural effusions
      122
   significance in sputum   13, 57
eosinophilic consolidation,
      differential diagnosis   48, 49
      Table 2.3
eosinophilia
   in allergic bronchitis   57
   in catarrhal children   131
ephedrine   79
erythema nodosum, in pulmonary
      sarcoidosis   143, 144-145
erythromycin, in treatment of
      pneumonia   50
ethambutol
   in treatment of tuberculosis
      99-100, 129
   toxic effects   100
exacerbations of chronic bronchitis
   antibiotic prophylaxis   62

see *also* chronic bronchitis
exercise provocation *see* asthma
expectorants in chronic bronchitis
   61
expiratory flow rate   32
   spirogram   32 Fig. 1.12
extrinsic asthma   71, 72, *see also*
      asthma
exudates, inflammatory,
      differentiation from transudates
      119-120, 122

farmers lung   136
FEV_1 (forced expiratory volume in
      one second)   23, 24
   in asthma   72, 73
   in chronic bronchitis   56, 57
   correlation with breath sounds
      25 Fig. 1.5
   normal value   33
   in pneumonia   43
fibroma, *see* mesothelioma
fibrosing alveolitis
   aetiology   135
   allergic alveolitis   136
      bird fancier's lung   136-137
      farmers lung   136
   crackles   29
   definition   135
   diagnosis
      pulmonary function   33, 136
      signs and symptoms   135-136
      X-ray   136
   dyspnoea   16, 19
   treatment   137
fibrosis   44
   and alveolitis   135
   complicating pneumonia   44
   after pulmonary sarcoidosis
      143-145
flucloxacillin, in treatment of
      pneumonia   50
forced expiratory time *see* breathing
      tests
forced expiratory volume in one
      second *see* FEV_1
fungal spores, and farmers lung
      136
fusidic acid, in treatment of lung
      abscess   51

gastro-oesophageal reflux

provoking laryngeal spasm   21
a cause of recurrent pneumonia
   45
gentamicin, in treatment of lung
   infections   51

Haemophilus influenzae
   in lung infections   37, 51
   in sputum   41, 57
haemoptysis   14–16
   in cancer of the lung   107
      relief by radiotherapy   118
   in fibrosis and bronchiectasis   44
   management   15, 16
   in tuberculosis   90
haemothorax, differentiation from
   haemorrhagic effusion   126
hamartoma   114
Heaf test   95
heart failure
   association with chronic
      bronchitis   59
   crackles and   29
hepatomegaly
   and lung cancer   110, 117
herpes zoster, and chest pain   22
hilar lymph nodes, in sarcoidosis
   143
histamine, in asthma   69, 70
hormones, in treatment of neoplastic
   effusions   130
Horners syndrome   110, 117
hospital admission, indications for
   airway obstruction in children
      132
   bird fancier's lung   137
   in pneumonia   49
   in pneumothorax   140
   in tuberculosis   101, 102
hydrocortisone *see also*
      corticosteroids
   in emergency treatment of asthma
      86
hypercalcaemia, in lung cancer
   110
hypercalcaemia, in sarcoidosis   143
hypersensitivity
   in catarrhal children   131
   tests
      in aspergillosis   76
      in asthma   73
hypertrophic osteoarthropathy, in

lung cancer   108
hyperventilation   18
hypnotherapy, in asthma   84
hyposensitization, in asthma   83–84
hypoxia
   bedside test for   30

immigrants
   tuberculosis in   89–92, 89
      Table 5.2
immune deficiency
   and recurrent infections   37, 45,
      134
   and catarrhal children   131
immunity to viral infections in
   children   131
Immunoglobulin A (IgA), and lung
   defences   35
Immunoglobulin E (IgE)   74, 131
immunosuppressive drugs, and
   pneumonia   36, 37
industrial dust, and lung cancer
   106
industrial injuries benefit, and
   mesothelioma   128
infection, defences and predisposing
   factors   35
   see also named diseases
influenza   11, 132
   virus as a cause of pneumonia   37
   vaccine in chronic bronchitis   62
Intal
   in asthma   80–81
   and chronic bronchitis   64
   effect on PEFR   33
   in recurrent respiratory illness in
      children   133
intestinal obstruction, in cystic
   fibrosis   134
ipratropium bromide *see*
   bronchodilators
isoniazid
   neuropathy   100
   prevention by pyridoxin   101
   in tuberculosis   98–100, 129
isoprenaline *see* bronchodilators

Klebsiella pneumoniae   39
   in sputum   41, 42
   treatment   51

kyphoscoliosis   39

laryngeal spasm   20, 76
Legionella pneumophila   37
lips, pursing a sign of airflow
    obstruction   31
lung, defences and factors
    predisposing to infection   35
lung cancer *see* cancer of the lung
lymphadenitis, and tuberculosis in
    immigrants   91
lymph nodes, and lung cancer   110
lymphocytes, in pleural effusions
    122, 127 Table 7.1

macrophages, alveolar, and lung
    defences   35
Mantoux test   95, 96
mast cell   70, 74, 80
mediastinal obstruction, in lung
    cancer   108, 110, 112, 118
mediastinoscopy in lung cancer
    113
Meigs' syndrome   125
mesothelioma   22, *see also*
    neoplastic effusions
  diffuse malignant   127–128
    and asbestos   127
    treatment   130
  localized (fibroma)   126
metastases   112, *see also* lung
    cancer, mesothelioma, pleural
    effusions
  in lung cancer   108, 117
  pleural   124, 130
middle lobe syndrome   15
miliary tuberculosis   93, *and see*
    tuberculosis
mitral stenosis and haemoptysis   15
'morning dipper'   72, *see also*
    asthma
mouldy hay, and farmers lung   136
mucus-secreting acini, and chronic
    bronchitis   54
mustine   130
mycetoma   15
Mycobacterium, see also
    tuberculosis, pleural effusions
  environmental   95
  tuberculosis   94, 100, 123, 124
mycoplasma
  in pneumonia   37, 40, *see also*

pneumonia
  diagnosis   42, 43
  treatment   50

neoplastic effusions   120, 124–125
  treatment   130
  see also mesothelioma, pleural
    effusions
neurological syndromes, and lung
    cancer   108
non bacterial pneumonia *see*
    pneumonia
noisy breathing   23–24, 72

occupational asthma   70, 77, *see*
    asthma
oestrogens, in treatment of cancer of
    the breast   130
oral contraceptives, inactivation by
    rifampicin   100
orciprenaline *see* bronchodilators
osteitis, tuberculous   91
oxygen treatment   *see named*
    diseases

pain, acute and chronic   21, 22
  and cancer of the lung   108,
    110–111, 118
  and inflammatory exudates
    119–120
  and neoplastic effusions and
    mesothelioma   126, 127, 130
  and pneumothorax   140
  and tuberculous pleurisy   124
parainfluenza virus   37, 132
PCO_2 and PO_2 *see* blood gases *and*
    named diseases
  in chronic respiratory failure   60
    Fig. 3.3, 68
peak expiratory flow rate *see* PEFR
percussion *see* clinical signs
pertussis, cough in   11
PEFR (peak expiratory flow rate)
  correlation with breath sounds
    23
  measurement and normal values
    33, 34 Table 1.1
  see also named diseases
penicillins   50, 62, 129
phenylbutazone   130
physiotherapy
  in chronic bronchitis   66

in lung infections   51–52
pigeon droppings, and bird fancier's
    lung   136
philocarpine iontophoresis   134
pleural effusions
    aetiology   119–120
    biopsy   123
    clinical signs   120
    differential diagnosis   123
    fluid, investigations of   122–123
    haemorrhagic   126
    postpneumonic   43–44
    Meigs' syndrome   125
    mesothelioma   126–128
    neoplastic, *see* neoplastic
        effusions
    purulent   126
    rheumatoid   125
    serous   123–125
    summary   127 Table 7.1
    systemic lupus erythematosus
        125
    treatment   128–129
    tuberculous pleurisy   124, 129
    tumours   126–128
    X-ray   120 Fig. 7.1, 121
pleural fluid *see* pleural effusions
pleural plaques   121
    and malignant tumours   122
pleural pressure, in pneumothorax
    139–141
pleural thickening   121, 128
pleurisy   21, 22, 39, 43, *see also*
    pleural effusions
pleurodesis, in pneumothorax   141
pneumococcus   37, 50
Pneumocystis carinii   42
pneumonia
    atypical   38
    bacterial   38
    classifications   37–38
    clinical features   38–40
    complications   43–44
        pleurisy   119, 123–124
    differential diagnosis   46–49, 49
        Table 2.3
    investigations
        serology   42–43
        sputum   41–42
        respiratory measurements   43
        X-ray   40–41
    lobar   37

and lung cancer   107
    pain   21
    recurrent   44–46
    suppurative   39
    treatment   49–52
        antibiotics   50–51
        hospitalization   49–50
        oxygen   51
        postpneumonic effusions
            128–129
    tuberculous   91
    viral and other non bacterial   35,
        37, 40, 123, 128–129
pneumonitis   38, *and see* pneumonia
pneumothorax, spontaneous
    dyspnoea   18
    pain   21
    pathogenesis   139
    recurrence   140
    risk associated with transpleural
        biopsy   113
    symptoms and signs   19, 140
    treatment   140–141
PO$_2$ see blood gases
polyarthritis and sarcoidosis
    144–145
polyarteritis and asthma   71, 78
polymorphs in pleural effusions
    127
postural drainage
    in chronic bronchitis   66
    in cystic fibrosis   134
    in pneumonia   52
precipitins in bird fancier's lung
    137
prednisone see corticosteroids
pregnancy, effect on asthma   77
Proteus in sputum   41, 42
Pseudomonas pyocyanea   42, 51
psittacosis   37, 40, 50
psychotherapy in asthma   84
pulmonary embolism   18
pulmonary infarction   21, 46, 49,
    see also named diseases
    serous effusions following   123,
        126
pulmonary oedema   19, 29, 75
pulmonary sarcoidosis *see also*
    sarcoidosis
    bronchial stenosis   144
    natural history   143–144
    treatment   144–145

pus in sputum 13, 14
pyogenic organisms *see named*
    organisms
    in pleural effusions 123
pyridoxin 101

Q fever 37

radioactive albumin, in diagnosis
    34
radioactive gas, in diagnosis 34
radiotherapy 114, 117–118
    and mesothelioma 130
râles *see* crackles
recurrent respiratory illness in
    children
    symptoms and signs 132
    treatment 132–133
    viral infections 131–132
    see also catarrhal children, cystic
        fibrosis
renal failure and sarcoidosis 143
respiratory failure in sarcoidosis
    144
    see also chronic respiratory
        failure
respiratory syncytial virus 37, 132
rheumatoid pleurisy 119, 122, 125
rhinovirus 132
rhonchi *see* wheezes
rickettsia 40, 50
rifampicin 99–100, 129
rimiterol *see* bronchodilators

serological tests in pneumonia 40,
    42–43, 45
serous effusions 123–125, *see also*
    pleural effusions
SLE, pleurisy and effusions in 125
smoking 53, 105, 114–117 *see also*
    cancer of the lung, chronic
    bronchitis
sodium cromoglycate *see* Intal
sputum
    blood stained 14
    culture 41–42, 42 Table 2.2
    retention 35
    smear 42, 57
    see also named *diseases*
squamous cell carcinomata 106,
    see also cancer of the lung
staphylococcus

infections 37, 39–41, 45, 50, 51,
    134
    in sputum 41, 42, 47
Streptococcus pneumoniae see also
    pneumococcus
    infections 37, 50
    in sputum 41, 42, 57
streptomycin 51, 101
stridor 12, 27
subphrenic abscess *see* abscess
surgery
    in cancer of the lung 117–118
    in extrapulmonary tuberculosis
        102
symptoms 11–23, *see also*
    individual *symptoms and named*
    diseases
systemic lupus erythematosus *see*
    pleural effusions *and* SLE

tall stature and pneumothorax 139
tension pneumothorax 139–140,
    see also pneumothorax
terbutaline *see* bronchodilators
tetracyclines 50, 62
theophylline
    in asthma 79–80
    in chronic bronchitis 64
thiotepa 130
thoracotomy 113, 117, 141
thrush, and corticosteroid aerosols
    82
Tietze's disease *see* costochondritis
tine test 95
tobacco 114–115, *see also* smoking
tonsillectomy 133
tracheobronchitis in smokers 11
transpleural needle biopsy 107,
    113
transudates
    causes 125–126
    differentiation from inflammatory
        exudates 119–120
tubercle bacilli *see Mycobacterium*
    tuberculosis
    in pleural fluid 123
tuberculin test 95–97
tuberculosis
    contacts, investigation of 96–97
    diagnostic tests 92–96
    haemoptysis 14, 15
    hospitalization 101

mortality   87, 88 Fig. 5.1
natural history   87–89
pain   21, 22
presentation   90–92
   unusual in immigrants   91–92,
   92 Table 5.1
prevention   97–98
treatment   98–103
X-ray, normal   90–91
tuberculous effusions   122
tuberculous pleurisy
   complications   128
   differential diagnosis   124, 126
   treatment   129–130
tuberculous pneumonia   91
tumours
   clubbing of fingers in   30
   intrabronchial   11, 14, 30
   pleural *see* pleural effusions
   silent   106, 107
   see also lung cancer *and*
      mesothelioma

urine, discoloration by rifampicin
   100
uveitis and sarcoidosis   143

vascular occlusion, pulmonary, tests
   for   34
viral infections   11, 37, 40, 43, *see
   also* pneumonia
   in children   131–133

water retention in lung cancer
   109–110
wheezes   25–28, *see also* clinical
   signs *and named diseases*

X-ray
   in acute lung infection   40–41
   in bronchiectasis   134
   in cancer of the lung   111 Fig. 6.1,
      112, 118
   in chronic bronchitis   57–58
   in emphysema   59
   in fibrosing alveolitis   136, 137
   in pleural effusions   120 Fig. 7.1,
      121 Fig. 7.2
   in pneumonia   38, 40, 41
   in pneumothorax   139, 140, 141
   in sarcoidosis   143, 144, 145
   in tuberculosis   90–91, 92, 93
      Figs. 5.3, 5.4, 96, 97

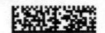